SAM EVANS

Past Pain

Recognizing, Resolving, and *Reversing* Neuroplastic Pain

* * *

Medical disclaimer

Content presented in this manuscript is not a substitute for professional medical advice, medical diagnosis, treatment, or therapy. It is presented and intended to provide general health and well-being information and solely for educational purposes. It should not be used as a substitute for medical care from a physician. Neither the author nor the publisher shall be liable or responsible for any loss or damage allegedly arising from any information or suggestion in this book.

Contents

1. Determine if this book is a valuable fit for you

Neuroplastic pain is real, it hurts, and it can be treated

Neuroplastic pain is a reversible brain-generated phenomenon. It is real, it hurts, but it can be treated. It has its genesis in the brain but is felt in the body. It causes immense physical suffering and mental anguish. I'm here to show how to treat it through simple, effective, and durable steps. By "simple," I mean small tasks or processes I can communicate to you, which you can practice yourself. By "effective," I mean treatments designed and tested by pain doctors and scientists and proven to reduce the magnitude of pain. This method is "durable" because it is designed to mesh with the realities of daily life and last for the long term. I know that these methods work because I have used them to recover from my own neuroplastic pain and helped others on their healing journey.

When I was diagnosed with chronic wrist pain, I didn't know what to do to make it better. Despite the input of some immensely helpful doctors, I was largely just stumbling around in the dark, going off-track, and getting lost. If something worked (or didn't), I had no idea why or how to maintain it for more than a day or two. It took me close to 10 years to heal from my neuroplastic wrist pain to the point of being pain-free. After that, I set out to understand why and hopefully speed up the process for others as a chronic pain educator and advocate. When you survive something as horrible as chronic pain, the least you can do is help others in their healing journey.

For you, neuroplastic pain symptoms may have initiated around a certain event, acute injury, or illness. For others —as in my case—there are no obvious organic sources or structural injury. This is because pain is a complex, biopsychosocial (bio-psycho-social) phenomenon. It's "biological," meaning pain can be a function of our physical health and genetic vulnerabilities. It's "psychological" in that it can be influenced by our minds and habituated by malleable brain signals, whereby temporary pain signals become permanent. And it's "social" because our environment and relationships can contribute to our pain story, for better or worse. We will untangle this complex biopsychosocial knot in more detail throughout the book.

A major theme of this guide is tackling the psychological aspect through a practice called "somatic tracking;" a psychological intervention that can make real, observable progress in your body. I'd like to invite you to engage with this psychological focus because we cannot always readily change our physical anatomy or orchestrate our external environment. It may feel a bit uncomfortable or downright confusing at first, so we'll break it down into small steps that you can apply to get unstuck for the long term.

Pain management is hard because you have to figure it out for yourself

This book is for people with neuroplastic pain who feel stuck in their pain management. You might have symptoms like back pain, neck pain, repetitive strain injury, fibromyalgia, migraines, irritable bowel syndrome, pelvic pain, or complex regional pain syndrome, and been told to just "learn to manage it" but were never given instructions on how to do so, what the ultimate destination is, or the process to get there. It's left to you to decipher all the pamphlets, books, podcasts, and pain management videos for yourself.

So why read this book when there are countless published works on chronic pain management? Do you really need another book?

To be honest, yes.

Many pain management techniques, books, and other materials follow a standard pattern. It goes something like this: an introduction to the author's background and expertise, anecdotes on previous patients' seemingly miraculous healing, the history of pain medicine, and details on the mind–body connection. Finally, we're given some information about how impactful cognitive behavioral therapy is, as well as more patient stories. These books largely showcase the author's expertise, get you excited about their idea, and then leave it up to you to handle the rest.

You read about it, and not much happens. You're left with a feeling of "great, now what's next?"

The issue with these books is they can be light on actionable steps for us to utilize. Conceptual knowledge has no value if we're unable to apply it, let alone understand the purpose of why we need to do it. It's not to say this material is bad; it's just not necessarily the best at delivering the exact steps on what to do to get better. That's where this book comes in.

The aim of this book is to leave you knowing what management is and how to effectively do it. This book has fulfilled its purpose if you can describe the end goal you would like to achieve with pain management and put treatments into practice to start feeling better. I'll show you how to incorporate them into your daily life for sustained success and to eliminate feelings of confusion and helplessness. You should never feel stuck or unclear on what to do next. Together, we'll make pain management work a little bit better.

Effective pain management isn't luck, you can design for it

Some people get lucky when it comes to pain management. You land on an amazing doctor, a miraculous surgery works, or you have a blinding revelation that turns your pain around 180 degrees. This is all wonderful when it happens, but what sets this material apart from others is the belief that successful pain management can be reliably designed for. It's not blind luck, a fluke, or some miraculous happenstance.

"Management" is the active steps we take to treat or reduce our pain. These activities usually occur outside and not necessarily within the walls of the doctor's office. "Management" can mean a plethora of things, such as physiotherapy, diet, exercise, medication, or conservative surgeries. But in this context, we'll define it as the psychological work we undertake to reduce neuroplastic pain symptoms. These steps will become routine, and this routine will be our pain management.

The proven effective treatment is called somatic tracking, and it will be the cornerstone of our work. Somatic tracking is a form of targeted mindfulness that rewires how our brain experiences pain. Pain is an experience, and we can reduce and even stop long-term neuroplastic pain sensations.

Before we jump headfirst into somatic tracking, this book explores how writing can help us express and resolve our pain-producing feelings. Then, we'll identify and work on reducing our pain triggers. Somatic tracking will be the capstone of our pain management system.

From my research, I've discovered that knowing the somatic tracking recipe isn't enough. Where the rubber hits the road is practicing it regularly, overcoming beginner barriers, and putting a plan in place so it is automatic, even if you are having a bad day or facing a flare-up. This is the hallmark of effective and durable pain management.

I realize that I've thrown around some terms that you may not have heard of before. And you probably have a bunch of questions, like: "What is somatic tracking exactly?", "Where on earth do I start with all this?" and "I don't understand what the 'psychological work' is?" We will cover these and more in detail throughout the following chapters.

There is an inherent leap of faith in starting anything new. I suggest reading this book in full to see the journey from start to finish. It will only take a few hours, and the concepts build on each other. You can then revisit sections to practice the skills. I've also included a brief appendix, a list of references, and some additional notes.

Where you might be coming from, and how this book can help you

Throughout your journey with neuroplastic pain, there are many paths that could have led you to this point. Ideally, a family physician, under guidance from a pain specialist or psychiatrist, has formally diagnosed you with a neuroplastic pain condition. Following diagnosis, you've developed a psychological-based treatment plan, but you need some guidance on how to execute the steps. If that sounds like you, amazing. However, pain can be episodic, so even if you've made some good headway, a flare-up or setback could nudge you to explore another perspective or equip another tool within your arsenal. Maybe you've got a good management process, but you need a reminder from this book to sustain your momentum.

The likely scenario is that you have arrived at this point because you've exhausted all options. A doctor has ruled out any obvious life-threatening or organic reason for your pain. If the pain was spurred by an initial injury, the site has long since "healed." You've done your own looking into the symptoms and, for a number of reasons, concluded your pain is indeed neuroplastic. Other people's case studies have resonated with you. You've spotted some evidence of neuroplasticity at work in your body. Maybe you've pieced together a treatment plan—even if you've never quite used that term yourself before.

You've got some grit. This work will help ease the burden, free up some brain space, and build on the foundation of your hard work.

Or maybe you're just not 100% sure. You've heard about this neuroplastic pain thing but need more time to get comfortable before ruling anything in or out. If so, I hope that seeing the end goal and steps along the way will help you on your quest.

For those who don't relate to the above, like a pain doctor, allied health worker, or carer—or if you're joining us from a completely different starting point—I hope this work will contribute to the neuroplastic pain community as a whole.

Let's be clear on who this book isn't for. If you're in the initial healing period of pain that is due to clear, acute tissue damage; for instance, a broken bone, hip replacement, sprain, infections, cancer-related pain, or nerve damage, then you will be better served by other means. While techniques in this book may be helpful, they don't have the same curative ability as for those suffering from the neuroplastic manifestation of chronic pain.

If the above doesn't align with your experience, I would respectfully suggest passing on this book. It will be a tough read, plus you'll probably find this work frustrating and not get very far. I would hate for you to waste your energy.

Once you've read the book, if you'd like to say hello, contact me at sam@pastpainbook.com.

Let's get started.

2. Why you might feel stuck in neuroplastic pain management and how to fix it

Pain management has poorly defined goals

Neuroplastic pain management rarely gives you a big goal to aim for. Nor does it specify the type of progress that you will make along the way. Without knowing what goal to achieve, you don't know how to focus your time and energy—and without stepping stones, you may get dissuaded and give up all too quickly. Worse still, it can stop you from outright trying. If it didn't work last time, why should you try again? You just spin your wheels.

With something like weight loss, it is easy to set goals and measure your progress. Stand on the scales and get a number. If the number is closer to your target, progress. If the number is higher, setback. When the number hits your target weight, mission accomplished. But how do you measure progress with pain? It feels so intangible because pain goals don't lend themselves to easy measurement—they are subjective. Significant improvements with pain can be made but is instead counted in terms of shifting thinking patterns, reclaimed responsibilities, improved emotions, and regained hobbies.

Without a quantifiable end goal, there cannot be any milestones guiding the way and pointing us in the right direction. Everything and nothing becomes a milestone. Consider if you want to take up running: Is a one-mile jog enough? Or do you need to run 10 miles per day? If you find yourself questioning the milestones, it is a sure sign the end goal is not clear. The milestones should be obvious and self-evident once the end goal is fixed in place. Yes, they may take some refining, but at least it isn't just a massive stab in the dark. There is no surer way of becoming disengaged than by taking random attempts at something. Even if one attempt turns out to be successful, how will you know?

Let's fix this now by setting a big goal. Take a typical pain-rating scale of zero to 10, where zero means no pain at all, and 10 is the worst pain imaginable and means you require heavy sedation in an intensive care unit. Working down the scale, it's likely you'd be reading this text from a maximum level of seven, where: "I am in pain all the time. It keeps me from doing most activities." Through applying the techniques in this book, our process is to reduce this high-tide mark of seven to, say, a goal of three, where the pain can be bothersome, but "I can ignore it most of the time." (We'll explain more evidence for this goal in Chapter 4.)

Having a permanent rating of zero is unachievable and can set you up for failure. We need to separate "zero neuroplastic pain" from the idea of "zero suffering." Even people who are otherwise completely healthy suffer from small pains dozens of times per day. This could include stiffness from sitting in an office chair too long, a minor back cramp, pangs of hunger, emotional hurt from challenging toddlers, or anger for being cut off in traffic. Total elimination is near impossible, but reduction via specific steps is highly probable.

Avoid pain management that has poorly defined goals. Let's start at seven out of ten and work our way down toward a three out of ten. This will be our North Star guiding us throughout the book.

Reading about pain won't necessarily get you out of pain

Many neuroplastic pain sufferers know all too well the frustration of being told to "read books on pain science" or "listen to good podcasts on chronic pain" only to not miraculously get better. What is the layperson supposed to do after reading all this cutting-edge pain neuroscience? There is a wealth of knowledge on how chronic pain works, but frustratingly little on how to get better during daily life.

There's a noticeable gap between textbook theory and practical application when it comes to finding relief. Pain doctors bring a wealth of knowledge and experience that can be truly transformative. However, effectively conveying this expertise in a way that's actionable and helpful to others presents a unique challenge. It's what some might call the "curse of knowledge." Starting off with dense neuroscience and complex journal articles often leaves beginners feeling overwhelmed and disoriented. It's understandable that this can lead to even more confusion instead of clarity.

However, there is something to be said about educating yourself on the causation of your pain—and we're entering territory that should be explored with your doctor. There are reported examples in academic literature of neuroplastic pain sufferers receiving relief from symptoms after educating themselves on neuroplastic pain. We'll pick this idea up in Chapter 3. But the learning outcome for now is, don't mistake consuming tons of pain information as equivalent to time spent in active, purposeful pain management.

You have to wade through filler information and vague case studies

Pain management material features boundless anecdotes and case study upon case study. While it is great to learn that "Jessica" recovered from pain overnight, rarely does it outline the exact steps she took in a manner that is repeatable for you and me. The other problem with personal case studies is that what people *think* worked and what *did* work are often vastly different. How can the rest of us achieve such enviable freedom from persistent pain? The reality is that neither Jessica nor the practitioner explained the exact steps that worked. It's like being asked to cook a new and highly complex pastry dessert recipe and only being shown the finished product. What steps am I supposed to follow?

I was fascinated by the question of why pain management doesn't seem to stick for good. I had to learn more and rapidly devoured every resource I could find: major books on the topic, YouTube lectures, courses, research papers, and podcasts. All of them had one major problem—they would devote less than 10% of their content to telling you how to take the steps to reduce or eliminate pain. Some content and information offered no steps whatsoever on how to reduce pain.

Pain management content is full of way too much filler material and not enough steps to actualize your own recovery. Pain management is a skill that can be communicated in the space of a few hours. Stick with pain management techniques that are to the point and give you the steps on what to do.

You may not see immediate benefits (but that's perfectly OK)

Somatic tracking is the meat of our pain management strategy. It's a targeted meditation and mental recalibration of your experience of pain (more in Chapters 4 and 7). This effective treatment has one major drawback: you need to practice it consistently, like you would with any new skill. This can risk being demotivating, especially when you don't see immediate results from the get-go.

People might try treatments like somatic tracking once or twice and then just give up. Life gets busy, and there are other things to do. It often feels like sacrificing the present to pay for the future, especially when the present is littered with more pressing obstacles, like grocery shopping or caring for children.

Neuroplastic pain treatments work, but why don't they always stick? It's probably the same reason why we don't go for a jog around the block three times per week or eat more vegetables instead of takeout. The reason is lifestyle. And it's a real piece of work. We are making genuine and verifiable progress when we go for our first half-mile jog, but it doesn't feel like progress if your aim is to run 10 miles. You don't see the instantaneous benefits after exercise, nor are you likely to see immediate benefits after attempting pain management treatment. The good news in both cases is that you are making real progress.

Neuroplastic pain management is a skill. As with any new skill, you typically see the most benefit after a period of dedicated, incremental practice. So don't be dissuaded or feel like you are stuck when you are only starting to learn the ropes.

Your takeaways from Chapter 2

Reducing neuroplastic pain is highly probable, but it's easy to feel stuck at first. It's a skill we can learn, so stack the odds in your favor by:

- having a single, clear goal to reduce pain from seven out of ten to three out of ten;
- avoiding getting overwhelmed with all the filler material and case studies;
- celebrating the first time you practiced active management steps. Remember, you've made important progress, even if you don't feel immediate results.

3. Knowing what neuroplastic pain looks like is the first recovery step

Neuroplastic pain is one of many unpleasant mind–body experiences

There is only one thing worse than chronic pain for most people: public speaking. Research shows that some fear it more than death.

Getting up in front of a crowd is no picnic. It's not the fact that talking is hard—many of us could speak at length unprompted about our hobbies, family, or that recent holiday we took. No, it's the sense of dread that comes with being under the public spotlight. This fear causes sensations in our bodies.

When the emcee calls you to the stage, your stomach feels sick, and your heart races. As you rise from your chair and make your way toward the lectern, your head gets dizzy, and your vision starts to disappear. You reach for the microphone with one shaky hand as the other clutches your notes in a death grip.

And then the nervous sweats start to happen. It's pretty hard to focus on nailing that opening line as a bead of sweat trickles down your forehead and onto your nose. Don't forget the shallow breathing and the squeaky voice, too. It's almost like you are gasping for air after every sentence.

I can count at least seven different physical reactions you can have when public speaking: shallow breathing, racing heart, sweating, stomach pains, dizziness, trembling, jaw clenching, and blushing. It can really be the worst.

Now, if my palms were getting sweaty, it would be misguided to try to reduce my sweating by applying antiperspirant deodorant to my hands. The antiperspirant will not reduce the dread and nervousness I feel about public speaking that is causing the sweating.

Alternatively, eating a healthy diet has obvious positive effects, but what impact would it have on improving my stomach sensations caused by my phobia of public speaking?

And how about the shaking? Why does standing up in front of others cause my muscles to involuntarily move and spasm against my will? How could the brain be so powerful?

Trying to fix these symptoms with lifestyle changes is like playing a game of whack-a-mole. Sure, I might get some temporary relief, but the underlying mechanical switches, servomotors, and puppetry are still in control. It's better to take a hammer to the power switch of the whack-a-mole machine (your thoughts) rather than the individual mole (the symptoms).

Maybe you sail through public speaking, and being in front of a crowd energizes you. You might get a massive adrenaline rush from being in the limelight. This, too, is due to your emotions.

Happy emotions change and shape our bodies, just as sad or anxious emotions can. It really is incredible that something as abstract and intangible as a thought can have very real, measurable, quantifiable, and repeatable effects on the way our body works. This is the mind–body connection. Our mental state can have big consequences on our muscles, digestion, and circulatory and nervous systems.

It is perfectly normal to find the mind–body connection unreal. The erroneous idea that our nonphysical thoughts and feelings are completely separate from our physical body built of atoms and chemicals has shaped Western thought. Once you start seeing the mind–body relationship at play in your daily life, it becomes difficult to ignore.

Emotions have also been shown to cause sensations like pain. For example, feeling scared about public speaking can make us sweaty, increase our heart rate, and slow digestion. It communicates that something is not right and something needs to change. Pain is another way our body communicates to our brain that something is not right and is just one of many unpleasant bodily experiences that happen daily.

You've probably already spotted ways that certain situations and feelings influence your body for better or worse. Understanding neuroplastic pain management hinges on recognizing the brain as the primary organ for pain perception.

Your brain is rewiring neurons to create pain signals without your consent

We've taken a big-picture look at how the way we feel in certain environments or situations can transform the way our body functions. This mind–body relationship is a critical framework, but how on earth does this relate to pain? For the remainder of this book, we will focus on just what this means for pain management.

We've used the term "neuroplastic pain" a number of times already, so in this section, we'll break the term down to figure out what's going on under the hood and how we can reverse engineer this into a recovery.

Let's start by defining "pain."

Chronic conditions aside, pain evokes words like "hurt," "danger," or "bad." It doesn't sound specific enough for our purposes, so we need a strong foundation and robust working definition of what pain is. For this, we'll leave it to the experts at the International Association for the Study of Pain (IASP), who describe pain as:

*"...an unpleasant sensory and emotional experience associated with, or resembling that associated with, actual or potential tissue damage."**

Beyond physical injury to our bodies, pain is a felt experience that is influenced by emotions and beliefs. The IASP has helped out here with these interpretations: "Pain is a very personal experience and usually influenced by biological, psychological, and social factors," "the concept of pain is something we learn during our life experience," and "pain is designed to be an adaptive role – to help us avoid bad situations. For some it may have an adverse effect on our way of life."

Let's talk about what pain isn't. It isn't something physical that we can touch, hold, or see—like a toxic molecule or a virus cell. We can't observe pain with a microscope or treat it directly with medication. One way of thinking about pain is like information transmitted from your cell phone to a cell tower. While we can touch, hold, and see the physical hardware of our phone, we cannot perceive the information flowing into and out of our phone with our five senses.

---

* See "The revised International Association for the Study of Pain definition of pain: concepts, challenges, and compromises." Raja, S. N., et al. 2020.

The most common pain experience for most people is acute pain. The name here can be misleading. Acute is not in reference to the seriousness of the pain; for example, an excruciating "10 out of 10" pain rating for a protruding broken bone. It doesn't matter whether it hurts a lot or not much at all. It can last for a few minutes or a few weeks. "Acute" is a reference to the time since the onset of pain. Classic examples are broken bones, lacerations, or strained muscles. Sporting injuries, workplace mishaps, and vehicle accidents are all common causes of acute pain. This form of pain normally resolves (gets better) once the injury site has healed. For example, a broken bone can take from 6–8 weeks to heal. Acute pain is usually done when healing is complete.

But what happens if the pain doesn't get better once an injury has healed? Or what if there was no injury to start with? It's time to explore the "neuroplastic" aspect of pain.[*]

Pain that persists in this manner happens when our pain signals build self-reinforcing neural connections. It's a negative feedback loop and can create an overactive pain system. Sufferers' brains have learned to experience stimuli in this way—all without our conscious control.[†] It can last for months to decades.

---

[*] Quick terminology note: Some medical professionals use the term "nociplastic pain" to describe neuroplastic pain.

[†] Several readers have reminded me of the "protective" nature of our neuroplastic symptoms. It can be a way of our body forcing us to slow down, say "no" to things, or reassess a certain situation.

The brain is always creating different pathways and habits, many of which are shaped by our emotions and cognition. The good news for us is that pain is just one of those plastic pathways that can be reshaped, dismantled, and reversed with the right effort. It does appear counter-intuitive because it's not the usual way we think about pain. Knowing how we can reverse engineer neuroplastic pain is an important step in designing our effective and durable pain management system.

So, how do I know if I have neuroplastic pain? In the next section, we will reflect on some questions about your journey to date. The more questions you answer in the affirmative, the more likely this book can help you.

How to know if your neuroplastic pain can be treated by this approach

We need to determine whether the neuroplastic pain or mind–body symptom you are suffering from is of the type that can be treated by this methodology. I do appreciate that neuroplastic pain doesn't always exist in isolation and can overlap or co-exist with other types of pain, and it might be challenging to tease apart. Therefore, I would recommend working through these questions with a doctor or healthcare provider.

Spend some time reading through the statements below. Write "agree" or "yes" next to the statements that reflect your experience, and "disagree" or "no" next to the ones that don't align with your journey to date.

1. In the past six months, have you had symptoms such as back pain, neck pain, repetitive strain injury, fibromyalgia, migraines, irritable bowel syndrome, pelvic pain, or complex regional pain syndrome?

2. If chronic pain was caused by an injury, has it continued for longer than six weeks, or after the soft tissue should have healed?

3. Did your chronic pain start without an obvious structural injury?

4. Did your symptoms start during a stressful time or event?

5. Do you have symptoms in other areas of your body? Do they appear to move around?

6. Has a doctor taken a detailed medical history and concluded no obvious organic cause?

7. Have you undergone testing and scans without an obvious organic cause for your pain? Tests could include blood tests, ultrasound, x-rays, CT scans, MRIs, or surgery.

8. Do your symptoms worsen or lessen during the day? Is your pain quality highly variable?

9. Do your symptoms worsen in stressful situations or anxious environments? Are they worse when anticipating a stressful situation?

10. Do your symptoms lessen in calm, relaxed environments (home vs. work) or while on holiday?

11. Do you have pain triggers that appear to have nothing to do with your body?

12. Do your symptoms reduce during sport, hobbies, and fun activities?

13. Are you a perfectionist? Do you have high expectations of yourself and others?

14. Are you driven to please others and put their well-being above yours?

15. Are you highly critical of yourself with unrelenting standards?

16. Do you have pessimistic tendencies or catastrophizing tendencies?

17. Does your pain worry you to the point that even anticipating pain is a major issue?

If you agreed with or answered "yes" to the majority of these questions, there is a strong likelihood of neuroplastic pain at play.

Some people might find reading these questions tough because they may trigger uncomfortable memories and force you to confront things you don't normally like to think about. Talking through these with a family member or close friend may help give you an external perspective.

The rest of this book is devoted to giving you actionable methods to alleviate these symptoms.

Your takeaways from Chapter 3

For people with neuroplastic pain, the brain, not the body, is the primary pain organ. It can cause painful sensations in the absence of injury or danger.

Use the above questions to identify if your symptoms are neuroplastic in nature. Did they start during an emotionally stressful time? Do you have pain triggers that appear independent of your body?

4. The science-backed steps we'll follow

Somatic tracking is the key treatment for neuroplastic chronic pain

In 2017, 44 sufferers of chronic back pain walked into a University of Colorado health clinic in Boulder, USA.[*] All of them had neuroplastic chronic pain averaging 4.10 on a 0–10.0 pain scale. And despite a range of medical investigations and interventions, all had been suffering for an average of 10 years. But after just one month of treatment with a pain psychologist, their pain reduced to an average of 1.18 on a 0–10.0 pain scale. The majority of patients described themselves as being pain-free or nearly pain-free. Yes, for many, the pain just stopped.

---

[*] It is well worth the time and effort to read the study in full, even if it is a little technical. See "Effect of Pain Reprocessing Therapy vs Placebo and Usual Care for Patients With Chronic Back Pain: A Randomized Clinical Trial." Ashar, Y. K. et al. 2022.

The "Boulder Back Pain Study" is a watershed moment for pain science. It is one of the most widely cited articles in its field. In this chapter, we will learn the same method detailed in the paper and how to translate it as we individually manage our own pain.

The main treatment method is called somatic tracking. It's like a form of targeted meditation or cognitive behavioral therapy. You may have heard of it as a component of the broader "Pain Reprocessing Therapy." We know from earlier chapters that neuroplastic pain is caused by maladaptive brain processes, and we can feel painful sensations despite not being in active danger. The crux of the approach is accepting that these misfiring signals are not an accurate sign of tissue damage. Treating this brain activity through the process of somatic tracking gave relief that lasted beyond the treatment.

This wasn't just a self-reported pain reduction either. Functional MRI scans were taken of patients' brains before and after. The results were clear: people who follow somatic tracking were literally restructuring their brains from experiencing chronic pain.

Neuroplastic pain is a reversible brain-generated phenomenon. What this means for you is that "something is wrong with my back" becomes "something is wrong with how my brain experiences pain." We will cover techniques in Chapters 5–7 to cement this mindset change and reverse neuroplastic pain.

Pain studies control one variable at a time— so should we

Before we leave the Boulder Back Pain Study, for now, there is one more major lesson we can take from it. Besides the somatic tracking treatment steps, there is another reason why it was so successful—and this one is not immediately obvious.

The chronic pain sufferers were specifically asked *not* to start any new treatments during the month-long somatic therapy regimen. This meant no strict diets, no changing medication, no different exercise routine, and certainly no use of aids like splints or braces. The purpose here was to hold other variables constant while testing the efficacy of somatic tracking.

Sure, having a healthy diet and exercising regularly is good—and essential for some—it's just not necessary for treating neuroplastic pain right now. What this means for you is that you can focus on the essential high-impact activities and address diet and exercise changes later. The philosophy is laser-focused on only selecting tasks that have a scientifically proven high probability of success and putting our time and energy there.

There are countless research papers, podcasts, books, and blogs presenting different treatment alternatives. Many of them are beneficial and complement the work in this book. But it's hard to make progress when you are constantly on alert for new treatment methods. The answer is to just put them on pause for now. There is plenty of time to address other self-improvements later. Give yourself permission to control one variable at a time.

The three-step method to stop maladaptive brain signals

This book has centered around two main ideas. The first is that your brain can cause very real bodily sensations like pain, cramps, dizziness, racing heart, and nausea. The second is that the underlying maladaptive (behaviors or responses that are harmful or ineffective) brain process can be rewired and ultimately changed for the better.

We can now switch gears from the problem of neuroplastic chronic pain to the solution. This shift allows us to start talking about treatment practices. Somatic tracking is usually undertaken as "talk therapy" with a skilled psychologist or counselor to guide you through the process. This book is a very different medium from face-to-face coaching. Therefore, we need to break down the treatment approach into three simple and repeatable steps that you can implement yourself.

Treating neuroplastic pain like this is an intimidating goal, but it doesn't need to be. Here are the actions distilled to an absolute minimum.

One: Emotional expression and awareness through writing

Being aware that our thoughts and feelings contribute to and sustain neuroplastic pain is the essential first step. We'll use writing activities to safely express and dismantle them (Chapter 5).

Two: Preventing and reducing neuroplastic symptom triggers

Identify the things that spark or exacerbate your pain. Learn techniques to eliminate or reduce these triggers (Chapter 6).

Three: Use somatic tracking on remaining pain sensations

Deliberately focusing on painful sensations in a safe, positive environment is the best method to achieve remission. This psychological intervention is proven to reduce pain signals from our misfiring brain (Chapter 7).

Pain management is an experiential skill, and you'll practice it over and over again. The three steps are very much "living and breathing," iterative, and evolve with time. To start with, you'll complete them in consecutive order, but with practice, you can skip around to what is most beneficial while avoiding dead ends and cul-de-sacs. This book will walk you through the skills in a way that is achievable in the short term and sustainable in the long term.

The goal of pain management is to maintain it with minimal effort

Applying pain management treatments from a book to your active life is a skill, but it's not meant to feel like a grueling chore. Yes, you will need to put in additional time and effort at the start, but this input is meant to be a temporary "short burst" of energy while you level up, not a long-term thing.

The first time you learned to drive a car, you were probably overwhelmed with all the pedals, gears, and controls—not to mention the road rules. It was exhausting, and you needed the expert guidance of a parent or instructor. Over time, shifting gears became second nature, as did navigating a busy intersection during peak-hour traffic.

At some point, you find that you've driven all the way to the grocery store without realizing it. Like learning to drive, successful pain management is achieved when you don't need to think twice about it—when it becomes second nature. The core techniques become automatic, requiring minimal effort to maintain. In practice, this means a significant reduction in symptoms to the point it does not impact or disrupt your daily life.

This skill-building process of pain management can feel like a process of trial and error. However, when you find an effective pain management approach that works for you, it brings immense clarity about the steps to take in your recovery. There is no more second-guessing or wondering if there is a "better way." This newfound clarity stops you from procrastinating and gives you the freedom to take action without constantly seeking different management resources. It gives you the ability to commit wholeheartedly.

Empty guarantees and the promises of miracles in healthcare often lead to disappointment and skepticism. My approach is to show you the most effective, evidence-based science and give you binary "yes-or-no" checkpoints along the way. If something isn't working, the benefit is knowing it quickly, not years down the track. It allows you to repurpose your effort into areas that do work. A big part of pain management is finding out what does not work, and the quicker, the better.

You will master neuroplastic pain treatment

It can be hard to start new practices and maintain changes when you don't get an immediate result or receive positive validation. Therefore, the following chapters have been designed to introduce small, real changes that make headway and lead to mastery. Because, like anything you master, you don't realize it until *after*, not during, the training itself.

Personally, I am always reminded of being a master of various skills when I need to teach someone else. It could be as simple as teaching a junior staff member how to do a technical process at work, showing a child how to draw with pencils, or helping a new sports club member navigate a training session. These are things we are so experienced in or over-familiar with that we forget they are even a skill. They happen intuitively and without conscious thought. It's all a form of mastery.

Reaching the master level of skill is one thing, but starting your chronic pain treatment journey is another. And if we don't notice changes until *after* we try something new, how do we know we are making progress in the right direction to begin with?

It's like setting out on a hike and being told that the next camp is "over there, to the right of us." How would we know when we had gone too far and missed it? Would we really know if we veered too far to the left? Or if it was 200 yards or 20 miles away?

You can see the problem with these kinds of treatment regimens. Therefore, it is far better to say that the camp is exactly 13 miles at 87 degrees to the east, that the terrain is a forest with light undergrowth, and that the camp contains open grass for setting up a tent and a freshwater river to collect water from.

Knowing the final location, travel distance, terrain, and obstacles in the way significantly increases the probability of successfully completing the journey.

Therefore, like the first tentative steps on a hike, during the initial treatment practice, you may not notice much at all. You *will* notice yourself crossing off specific progress steps along the way. Each step is designed as a quick win.

Use small, quick wins to level up

Quick wins are important because they show achievement and are an objective measure of progress toward mastery. We will use quick wins in our chronic pain recovery.

So, what is a quick win?

A quick win can be implemented by a newcomer (non-master) faster than other options or solutions. But beyond implementation speed, quick wins must have a high probability of success. For example, if we were starting an exercise program, 20 push-ups may be a great goal, but it is not in the quick-win category as it has a high probability of failure for a beginner. Simplifying 20 push-ups into a quick win doesn't necessarily mean reducing the target to just one push-up, either. Instead, a quick win would be putting on some gym clothes and doing five minutes of warm-up stretches.

Therefore, they must have a positive impact on your progress and keep the momentum going. This progress does not need to be majorly profound or earth-shattering; it just has to be a little bit better than yesterday's standard. Quick wins are your standard, not someone else's—

especially not another person who is more able-bodied than you or who has been practicing for a lot longer.

The opposite of a quick win is a setback. Setbacks can be deflating when they inevitably occur. Therefore, quick wins in this book are designed to be reversible if they don't work out as planned. This eliminates the hesitance or resistance to getting started. If something you try flops completely, the consequence is minor and can easily be undone.

The final thing about quick wins is that they must be celebrated. Seriously. It may seem trivial, but reminding yourself that you are powerful, capable, safe, and in control is important. Tell your partner, housemate, pet, or, better still, yourself. Not celebrating is a sure sign of perfectionism at play, as is the mindset of "I will only celebrate after I've achieved my massive final goal."

Quick wins are essential for keeping your recovery moving forward in the right direction, especially during the early stages when progress may be hard to notice. Without acknowledging your progress and steps forward, the tendency is to focus on your losses or setbacks. This can lead to frustration and ultimately lead to you giving up. It's like uprooting a sapling that hasn't grown more than an inch high only to discover its roots deeply embedded into the ground.

Get in touch with your health practitioner to make sure nothing has been overlooked

Decoupling pain sensations from an organic cause is a big mindset change that you will keep revisiting throughout your path to pain management mastery. To start, you need to get in touch with your health practitioner. The purpose of this is to:

---

1. Rule out any obvious, life-threatening, or organic sources of pain if you haven't already.

Benefit: This gets you off the hamster wheel of endless scans and tests that bring the focus back to your body, not how your mind experiences pain.

2. Communicate your neuroplastic pain management plan and state that you would like to take a mind–body approach with somatic therapy.

Doctors may be more familiar with a "psychophysiological disorder," "central sensitization disorder," or "psychosomatic" approach to pain management.

Benefit: Get clarity by verbalizing your plans to a professional for appraisal.

3. Find out if their experience with pain is a good fit with your management strategy.

Benefit: Find a medical expert you can regularly check in with and help with your concerns.

Speaking with a family physician means you need to trust their expertise. If they have ruled out serious acute problems or are unable to explain your pain from physical ailments, then great! Generally speaking, this is a very good thing to ensure there are no critical issues like a fractured vertebra or tumor. So, unexplained pain is a good thing for chronic pain sufferers.

Therefore, stop asking your doctor for one more test or another scan. Stop doubting the results. Chronic pain feeds off these anxieties and the need to do "just one more test." Instead, here's a script you can use to build consensus with your treating doctor (quick heads-up: the term "chronic pain" can mean a lot of different things to both patients and healthcare providers, so we'll substitute it for "psychosomatic disorder" as it flags with our doctor that we'd like to explore a mind–body approach):

You: "Hello, doctor."

Doctor: "Hi, how can I help you today?"

You: "We've been investigating what's causing my [insert neuroplastic pain symptom here] for quite a while now. All the x-rays, MRIs, and tests I've done have come up clear. I wonder if my [symptom] could be caused and sustained by unresolved emotions or stressors?"

Doctor: "Umm... OK. What do you mean?"

You: "I've noticed that my [symptom] gets worse when I am anxious or stressed [insert other triggers here]. Could this be a neuro-plastic or psychosomatic disorder? How can we investigate this together?"

You've now cleared the air with your treating doctor. All it took was a 15-minute appointment to short-circuit the treadmill of endless tests and scans. Once an organic cause has been ruled out by medical professionals, you need to cease and desist from the idea that your muscles, bones, nerves, and tendons are the problem.

Your takeaways from Chapter 4

Neuroplastic pain is brain signaling that produces painful sensations. The healing approach is to both reduce and counter this brain activity.

Master the three-step method for managing neuroplastic pain: express emotions, identify triggers, and use somatic tracking techniques.

Pain management is an experiential skill that you will master. You don't notice mastery until long after the training, so it's important to work with and celebrate quick wins to show real progress along the way.

Focus on controlling one variable at a time for effective pain management, just like in the Boulder Back Pain Study.

Communicate with healthcare providers to rule out organic causes of pain and align treatment strategies for effective management.

5. Writing reduces the severity of neuroplastic symptoms

Writing is the first active task of pain management

Your brain is abuzz with all sorts of anxious thoughts, feelings, and sensations. And this is perfectly normal—it's what a brain does. But, as we've seen in Chapter 3, our feelings can get out of control and cause physical pain. Therefore, in this chapter, we will utilize writing as a tool to organize our thoughts, get them out of our head, and expose them for what they are. In Chapter 6, we will explore how organized thoughts reveal patterns and evidence for chronic pain triggers, which can then be minimized. Armed with our newfound knowledge, in Chapter 7, we will explore how to soften pain experiences with somatic tracking.

Writing is an imperfect replacement for working with another person, like a counselor or psychologist, who can point out our blind spots or probe false assumptions. It lets you "see" your emotions and feelings, potentially for the first time. The aim is to understand your unconscious thoughts on pain and communicate this understanding to your conscious self. It's a vital feedback loop to challenge incorrect assumptions and advance recovery.

Writing our thoughts down is a proven method to reduce the symptoms of trauma, PTSD, anxiety, depression, stress, and, yes, neuroplastic pain. But the process of "writing" feels ambiguous; what exactly are we supposed to do during an expressive writing session? This chapter explains not only what you will be doing during these sessions but the science behind why it is effective.

Writing treats neuroplastic pain by expressing and accepting difficult emotions

To better understand the mechanics of how and why writing is so powerful, we will refer to a number of recent studies[*] that have employed writing as a tool for enabling emotional awareness and expression. Sufferers in these studies had neuroplastic symptoms from fibromyalgia, pain, irritable bowel syndrome, fatigue, anxiety, and depression.

---

[*] For the full studies, see *Bibliography* entries under a.) Graham, J. E., et al. 2008; b.) Hsu, M. C., et al. 2010; c.) Lumley, M. A., & Schubiner, H. 2019; d.) Carty, J. M. et al. 2019; and e.) Yarns, B. C., et al. 2020.

Each study looked at writing as a component of treating neuroplastic symptoms. There were some minor differences in methodology; some patients were offered cognitive behavioral therapy, others were given more education about pain, some treatment plans lasted weeks, while others went on for months. Despite this, the results were clear: voicing our emotions in writing reduces neuroplastic pain symptoms.

Understanding that neuroplastic pain symptoms are caused by unmodulated brain signals, the rationale is that stressful thoughts and conflicting emotions exacerbate these symptoms. By fostering emotional awareness and expression through writing, it becomes possible to modify and reverse these signals.

The hard part is embracing these negative emotions to start with. It took me a while to be comfortable enough to experiment and play with them. When feelings are on paper, they do not look as scary and terrifying as they do in our minds. We can quite literally take a step back to give us some much-needed space between our emotions and pain sensations.

Listing our immaterial thoughts on physical paper has meant that somewhere between our brain and the pen tip, we are forced to both organize our ideas and articulate them clearly. But that's not all. Writing means we have also applied a filter, criticism, and appraisal of our thoughts.

The long-term benefit of mastering this writing activity is being able to focus on the important factors that influence our pain while ignoring all the background noise. After all, understanding something is the first step in overcoming it. How else will you know where to spend your precious time when we cover managing triggers and somatic tracking in later chapters?

What should I write about?

You will write about three main areas:

1. The event that initiated your pain.
2. Things that keep sustaining it.
3. Times when you were not in pain (we'll call this counter-evidence).

Start with simple events at face value. List the first things that come to your mind.

An **event that initiated your pain** could be a sudden cause—like the twisting of a knee at work that has blown out to chronic pain. Initiation could be gradual, like the inevitable worsening of neck pain into chronic pain during your master's studies at university. For both cases, writing helps you understand the broader emotional context and your feelings at the time when you first noticed the pain. You see things you were unable to observe at the time of injury.

Regardless of how things got started, there are **events that fuel the pain and keep it going**. This could be desk work in your office that arouses your back pain, or physical activities and postures like sitting, bending, and twisting. Alternatively, it could be certain people in your life, such as overbearing in-laws or pestering co-workers, who cause tension headaches (social environments). The most challenging to identify is your own thought process or emotions—such as focusing on the pain the moment you wake up. Physical activities, social environments, and emotions trigger and sustain pain. We need to discover what they are by writing them down.

The final thing to write about is **counter-evidence of times you are not in pain**. Why does my neck hurt at work but not when I am outside gardening? Why don't I notice my back pain when I am play-wrestling with my grandkids? Why do my headaches stop on weekends or during holidays?

As you start writing, you may observe patterns: certain people, places, events, responsibilities, emotions, and feelings keep appearing; a set time of day, the exact name and description of a feeling, or the person who may be causing this. With time, these will crystalize into a trigger or cue that brings about the pain (Chapter 6).

Writing is work, and it will take time and energy. But think of it as a "short burst of energy." You are not meant to sustain it for years on end, but rather a few weeks of dedicated work.* There is no need to spend decades digging into the very depths of your psyche to unearth long-suppressed emotions or desires that would make Sigmund Freud blush. You are supposed to outgrow the writing exercise as you level up and master understanding your thoughts and feelings.

Write for 10 minutes in the morning before your daily routine

You'll need 10 minutes of time in the morning to complete your writing task from start to finish. This is non-negotiable, as it's when your brain is at its sharpest, and it sets the tone for the day.

Mark Twain summarized how to tackle writing like it's a chore: "If it's your job to eat a frog, it's best to do it first thing in the morning. And if it's your job to eat two frogs, it's best to eat the biggest one first." Translation: do the most uncomfortable task first.

Frogs are slimy, wriggly, and unpalatable, so if you have to eat one, it's best to tuck in as fast as possible. Don't think twice—just gulp it down. Your "frog" is a writing task. It's something that you have zero motivation for and are likely to procrastinate on for the rest of the day. You don't want to do it, but you need to do it.

---

* By all means keep up the practice in the long term if you find it beneficial. Some pain sufferers describe writing as a healthy daily habit—like working out and eating right—it's a long-term lifestyle change.

You may not think you have a routine, but you do. It could look something like this: Lie in bed scrolling on your phone until you are bored. Get up and make breakfast while watching television. Have a shower. Come back to the television and scroll your phone. Sure, it might not look like a routine, but, by definition, it is a routine.

Or maybe you are at the other end of the spectrum. Your alarm goes off at 6:00 AM on the dot. You are showered and dressed by 6:25 AM. You finish breakfast by 6:40 AM to make a mad dash down the block to catch the 6:55 AM bus to work.

It goes without saying that your writing time has to be undisturbed. You cannot check your phone, social media, or emails before or during this 10-minute session. They will weigh on your mind and contribute to pain-induced stress.

So, whatever your routine looks like, structuring it to include 10 minutes of writing is a must.* You can make it task-based scheduling: Write immediately after having my breakfast, but before I sit down with a coffee to watch TV. Or time-based scheduling: Write between 6:10 AM and 6:20 AM. This kind of schedule has a high proba-

---

* If doing this in the morning really doesn't work for you, try writing in the evening after a full day. Some people use the evening time as an outlet and more of a brain dump to think of things that triggered or bothered them from that day (rather than the previous day).

bility of success and makes tangible progress in moving your recovery forward—it's a quick win.

Use pen and paper, and put your devices in another room

Before you write your thoughts down, you'll need some tools to do the job properly and keep you grounded in this treatment activity. When we think of writing equipment, we first think of our laptop or phone. This is our note-taking tool of choice for most other writing activities, but for this task, electronic devices are not allowed.[*]

Electronic devices are a magnet for distraction and multitasking. Family members who see us chipping away on a laptop can interpret that we are just killing some idle time on social media. This is an ambiguous signal that you are working on a low-value task that invites disturbance.

Therefore, get off your computer and pick up a pen and some paper. A dedicated paper notebook might feel less disorganized and chaotic than loose scraps of paper.[†]

---

[*] For some people, the only option for writing is an electronic device. If this is you, try some useful strategies to reduce disruption from people in your household: include a "do not disturb sign," or set your phone on airplane mode or turn off the wi-fi to avoid multitasking.

[†] I do know of people who prefer writing on scrap paper so they can immediately scrunch it up and throw away their finished writing. This can be an act of "letting go" of difficult emotions. Experiment and see what works for you.

Another advantage of a paper notebook is that your writing, thoughts, and feelings are contained in a separate object. You can literally park your thoughts to one side and tuck them away back on the shelf or in your bag. Therefore, don't use this notebook for anything else, like shopping lists or to-do tasks.

Now that you have your tools—a notebook and a pen—put them in a nice room or space that's dedicated to writing only. Make sure it is well lit. Keep some indoor plants. Light a candle or play some music if it helps you concentrate. The only condition of this room is that it cannot contain a laptop, PC monitor, or phone. Yes, this is hard to achieve for those of us living in cozier spaces, so, as a minimum, get your computer and phone out of reach and visual sight.

If you're trying to write in a busy household, it just invites interference. It's totally logical for a partner or housemate to think, "You can't be doing anything important, so now is a good time for me to interrupt with my question about dinner plans for next Friday." Having a physical notebook open at a secluded table is a signal to your partner or family that you are working on a high-value task: "Do not disturb." The first week of your writing routine will be an opportunity to practice assertiveness in asking for space and time from your household (I guarantee it).

If all else fails, and writing at home just doesn't work for you, change your environment; it's been proven to help with creativity and forming new ideas. Go to a nice coffee shop, park, or public space. Working in a space with strangers can produce a sense of accountability—there are other people around me, so I should get cracking with my work. This is known as "body doubling" and has seen a rise in popularity as we've shifted more to virtual or remote work.

Will you ever read this journal again? Will your romantic partner "discover" it and pore lovingly over every last sentence? Will the film rights be sold to Hollywood for a multi-million-dollar sum? Probably not. The aim of journaling isn't to leave an autobiographical manuscript for future generations, but rather to bring any stressors or unconscious worries to light. If you are writing for someone else or building a personal legacy, you will instinctively filter out parts of your thinking or censor certain emotions, which leads to procrastination, spinning your wheels, and generally getting stuck. We're not building legacies here, so don't get caught thinking this way.

Write to identify past events that initiated your pain

Using writing to identify your inner emotional state or external environment at the initiation of pain reveals triggers (Chapter 6) and a way forward with treatment (Chapter 7). Our focus for this section is on past events, not current or future situations.

Our physical pain is like a lightning rod in an emotional electrical storm. We can hear and see the crackling of electricity overhead. And then, boom! Emotional feelings get encoded as real physical pain. So, what was the lightning strike that caused your pain to start? You may have had a buildup of frustrations with your partner for years. Suddenly, you experienced back pain just as they were about to leave for a week-long business trip.

It could be less obvious and more gradual in others. Studying at university brings about a lot of emotions with the pressure of needing to get high grades, the loneliness of being in a different city from friends and family, and having to juggle part-time work to make ends meet as a student. Ever so slowly, tension headaches start to develop. At first, it's just a one-off, but as the years roll by and the academic stakes are amplified, headaches appear like clockwork when an assignment is due.

The above examples are fairly obvious to an external reader. But in the heat of the moment and in the midst of suffering, it is very hard to notice the link or underlying pattern. This is the value of writing—it helps us see things in a more objective light as if we were reading someone else's case study.

We will use the 10-minute writing exercises to get you to a more organized and objective point of view. Feel free to work through these points at your own pace. As a guide, one point on the list per day will get you there in three weeks.

When you first noticed pain

What was life like in the weeks before your pain?

What date and time of day were you first aware of your pain?

Was there an obvious cause or accident, or did it just appear out of nowhere?

What was your reaction?

Your physical body

Describe your energy levels, sleep patterns, and physical health in the days prior to the onset of pain.

What types of exercise were you doing at the time?

If you found some relief when pain first occurred, what was it?

Do you have other symptoms? What are they?

What happened the first time you went to a doctor to explain your symptoms?

Environmental and physical surrounds

What physical environment were you in the day you were first aware of your pain?

Did you have a major life event? Moving town, moving house, new job?

What did you do physically to respond to your pain? For example, quitting a job, buying support equipment, less/more exercise?

Social life

What social environment were you in the day you first noticed pain?

What external responsibilities did you have during the week prior to the pain?

Did you have a major life event? For example, a

new relationship, break-up, caring for a sick relative, finishing school or college?

Were there changes in your friendship group? Too many friends to keep up with? Not enough?

Your personality and emotions

How would you describe your personality in your life up to encountering pain?

List the major emotions you were experiencing in the weeks prior to the pain.

What other meaning do you associate with your pain? This could be spiritual or symbolic.

If your pain is telling you a message, what would it be?

What other things were on your mind at the time of pain?

Each question presents a lot of material to write on in just 10 minutes. And this is intentional, so you don't over-think it. Just write down everything that comes to mind unfiltered. Having constraints and a deadline helps to focus your thinking as you practice this emotional aware-ness and expression therapy.

Finally, to reiterate, all these questions relate to the start of pain or when you first noticed it. It is helpful to attach a calendar date to it so your writing doesn't drift forward in time to your present feelings toward pain. If you can't remember an exact date, be as specific as you can about the weeks or months immediately prior to your pain.

Write to identify the things that currently sustain your pain

The last section was exclusively writing about what happened on or around the onset of pain. Questions were intentionally fixed in the past and disproportionately focused on thoughts, emotions, social life, and feelings. And there was a reason for this spotlight on feelings. The majority of unpleasant or painful things that happen to us are mental processes, like pessimistic thoughts, anxious worries, relational hurt, or general cognitive exhaustion. This suffering and pain can happen dozens of times per day.

Contrast that with how often we suffer from a physical injury like a stubbed toe or papercut; if we are really unlucky, maybe once per week, if at all. The vast majority of our suffering is mental. It happens within, not outside, the walls of our skull. This means that most of the unpleasant things that happen to us don't result from actual physical bodily harm.

Therefore, the more we organize our feelings about the way we experience pain, the better we can implement tools to reduce it. This section will ask you to be precise about how you respond to pain in the here and now. We'll introduce the definition of a "flare-up"—a period of time when your pain was greater than usual and made you stop to notice and think about it; it wasn't just part of the background noise.

This is an intentional shift in gears from the previous section, as we start to find unconscious patterns or repeated habits around pain flare-ups, how you notice them, and your response. In Chapter 6, we will codify these patterns as triggers, but this isn't the objective here; we're still in the realm of getting some scribbles down on paper.

You'll need to keep spending 10 minutes doing your morning writing routine to answer these. The only exception is if you are able to do your writing during or immediately after an actual flare-up (the insight here would be unparalleled).

Your beliefs about pain

What do you think about your pain now?

What day and time did your last flare-up start? (Or when do you usually notice your pain?)

How did you react to your chronic pain during your most recent flare-up? What thoughts did you have, and what behaviors and actions did you take?

Will your pain ever get better?

Environmental

If I could change anything about my employment situation, what would it be?

What changes would I like to make about my home environment?

Social

What social responsibilities should I have eliminated a long time ago?

If I could make any changes to my social group, what would it be?

What family members do I need to move away from, and what family members do I need to reconnect with?

What reasonable criticism do my family and friends have about how I deal with pain?

Personality

How do I react to other forms of pain in my life?

What would your family say are your major personality traits?

Do you feel like something is missing from this list, but you can't put your finger on it? Feel free to ask family members, housemates, or trusted work friends about some of these questions. This is where the external perspective is useful.

Get tangible counter-evidence to demonstrate the plasticity of pain

Chronic pain can make you afraid of recurrence, and it puts you on high alert all the time. Reduce this fear with counter-evidence of times when your pain has decreased in magnitude. This exercise helps erode your hypersensitivity to pain.

The key feature of neuroplastic pain that we will be targeting is the fact that it changes in magnitude. Sometimes it's really bad, other times it's manageable, and sometimes it even momentarily disappears. The pattern here is that it is non-consistent. And this is important.

An example might be if I have terrible wrist pain and can hardly bear operating a cash register or scanning item barcodes at work, yet I can happily enjoy knitting, crocheting, and sewing for hours on end at home with minimal pain. This is an important data point as it shows the inconsistency of pain. Why would our chronic pain suddenly "flare-up" or "calm down" with no changes in biomechanical movements?

Personally, I was struck by the fact my pain reduced slightly while on holidays or on weekends. The problem was that it took me years to put two and two together. Once I did, it was easily the biggest insight into just how the brain impacts pain because it showed me there was a mechanism for reduction.

People who have been in pain for a long time develop a negativity bias, whereby they only identify and pick up on negative occurrences of bodily sensations. This means we get blinded to positive experiences, sensations, and good times when the pain is reduced. Effort, via applied writing, is required to get counter-evidence and reduce this. Here are some questions to get you started:

- What works for reducing pain? (Or flip the question and ask what makes it worse.)

- In what environment do I feel the most free of pain? Home, sports field, shopping center, vacation, in the office?

- If sitting/lifting/twisting/standing/sleeping usually causes pain, are there times I have sat/lifted/twisted/stood/slept without pain?

- What times am I "in the flow" and hours seem to just rush by?

- Do I notice the pain when I play sports?

- Are there times I've been so absorbed in a hobby that I don't notice my pain?

- What am I doing the instant I notice that

I am not in pain? What about the exact moment before that?

• Do different actions with the same affected body part have different pain levels? (For example, typing causes wrist weakness, yet opening a tight jar lid doesn't. Or sitting at work is painful, yet moving or twisting your back isn't?)

• Are there certain people I am around that cause pain to reduce?

• Is my pain worse or better at different times of the day?

• Did the pain start without any physical changes to my body?

Your brain has now seen important evidence of when your pain reduced in magnitude.

Inconsistencies in your pain help show us that it is at least partially influenced by emotional occurrences, social situations, and environment, and not necessarily the physical condition of your body.

Before we move on to the next chapter, remember this writing is all a data point gathering exercise. Some data points are good, some are bad, and many are moderately useful. When you get enough of them, you will be able to sort them into patterns. Typically, this is achievable in four weeks of practice; however, some people may need less time, and others benefit from making this a more permanent habit.

This chapter was intense. We've seen that our physical environment, social group, emotional state, and own personal attitudes create and maintain pain. Writing has allowed us to safely express these emotions and use them to find patterns about triggers.

Writing might be challenging

Dealing with negative emotions and thoughts is hard. It's easy to be put off by this and shy away from even starting. This will be the biggest barrier to gaining the immense benefits of writing. One strategy to try is to tell yourself that it could be uncomfortable for the first few moments, but the good news is that this expressive writing does help in reducing symptoms.

Reflective writing and introspection do not come naturally to some, and there are few of us who would intentionally sit down and dedicate time to fleshing out our thoughts and feelings. So don't be dissuaded if you cannot immediately communicate your thoughts in writing like a pro.

One messy handwritten paragraph is a quick win

Completing a scheduled 10-minute writing session qualifies as a quick win. We know that writing is a proven antidote to pain, and if we practice it, even for just one messy paragraph, this is moving in the direction of the pain management we want.

By all means, celebrate it with a coffee, a walk, or a few minutes of social media. Some people underestimate this and dismiss it as not much to be proud of. But not you; you know much better. A win in pain management is massive.

Don't worry if what you have put on paper doesn't contain anything immediately insightful; it's just an initial data point, and it's impossible to fit a trend into a single bit of information. Therefore, identifying and dismantling the long-term patterns and triggers of your pain needs numerous data points. String a few daily quick wins together to reach an end-of-week milestone. Build out a few weeks into a month to start cementing this positive habit. Before you know it, you will have 20+ data points in your catalog of messy handwritten notes.

Your takeaways from Chapter 5

Expressive writing is a powerful tool to reduce neuroplastic pain symptoms by organizing thoughts and exposing underlying triggers. Writing helps identify emotional patterns and triggers, paving the way for targeted treatment.

Embrace discomfort and commit to daily 10-minute writing exercises to explore the initiation of pain, factors sustaining it, and moments of pain relief.

Cultivate counter-evidence of pain reduction to highlight the plasticity of pain and mitigate fear of recurrence.

6. Identify and then decrease what triggers your pain

The last chapter was the first of three big chunks of theory and has set you on course for a major behavior change: four weeks of daily writing practice. I recommend against setting this book down until you are ready to move on in four weeks' time because knowing the remaining steps of pain management helps to answer the questions: "Why are we doing this again?" and "How does this actually help me?"

So, why are we doing this? The aim of the writing activity isn't to leave an autobiographical tome for future great-grandchildren. Instead, it will help you see longer-term patterns and gain the emotional awareness you can only get from "zooming out" and constructing your thoughts in text.

This chapter clocks up gains by finding what triggers your pain and making a plan to reduce it. It's just like knowing that you are allergic to peanuts (the trigger) can stop hives, swelling, or anaphylaxis. Or how the "ping" of a phone notification can trigger you down an hour-long social media spiral. Silencing our phones or avoiding peanuts can stop the trigger and resulting negative outcomes. Our response to neuroplastic pain has much in common.

A trigger starts an automatic process

Our whole life is a wave of prompts, nudges, pushes, and pulls in one direction or another. Some are fairly weak, like a social media advertisement that triggers you to think about a certain product and maybe click through to the product page. Others are more important, like the wail of a police siren or the smell of something burning on your stovetop. We will classify these as "triggers" because they cause us to take action or change direction. A trigger initiates a process.

A process is a predefined series of events or patterns that happen automatically. Processes are hard to spot because many of them are second nature, which is the main reason for the writing task in Chapter 5. When a trigger happens, like a yellow traffic light changing to red, we don't go back to the drawing board and figure out the exact distance to the intersection and what steps we need to take to apply the brakes. It is automatic. We instinctively slow down and stop at the traffic light without a second thought. Processes are good because they free up brain space and take less cognitive energy in the long term.

The more a process happens, the more solidified it becomes. You shift from having to consciously think, concentrate, and work hard to make it happen to not giving it a second thought. This is also how habits are formed. It's easiest to think about physical processes, like developing muscle memory during a football training drill, sitting on the couch to watch a TV series immediately after dinner, or knitting a sweater row after row. These are things we can see, and we have the ability to shape our environment, time, and money to participate in them.

Our feelings and emotional experiences are similarly shaped by this trigger-process relationship. Mental triggers based on "feelings" can be hard to spot because they lack tangible external references, unlike those in the physical world. Pain is an example of an automatic process that can be triggered and brought to our attention.

Learn to spot triggers

When we link this back to pain management, the most straightforward approach and solution to pain is eliminating negative triggers. By removing the starter's gun, we can eliminate the race altogether. Stopping the input means there is no output, regardless of whatever black box processing goes on in between. No trigger equals no pain, right?

While this would be a wonderful outcome, it's a big undertaking. We're putting the cart before the horse. Instead, we'll see that identifying some triggers and breaking them down into the tiniest chunks imaginable is not only an easy way to get a quick win but also makes headway to breaking the trigger-process cycle. The goal here is to become more adept at recognizing your neuro-plastic pain triggers. Recognition of pain is what helps us to undertake effective somatic therapy later in Chapter 7.

Find things that make you aware of your pain

We've spoken about this idea of "awareness" a lot already, so it's long overdue to define it. Awareness simply means being able to describe how something feels. A simple exercise to check whether we have an awareness of something is to scan through our six senses one by one: sight, sound, smell, taste, touch, and proprioception.* (Proprioception is the sense of the movement of our muscles and body in space.)

Delving headfirst into our pain triggers can be a roller coaster of feelings. However, there is an upside to noticing a trigger. This can be a valuable chance to

---

*   I'd like to invite you to "dial-up" your curiosity of this sense. People have found that yoga, Pilates, and breathing exercises are helpful ways of getting comfortable with tuning into your body and engaging your proprioception.

actively describe what it is like. This newfound knowledge will be invaluable for reducing the impact of our neuroplastic pain.

Start by identifying external pain triggers

We will now reconfigure our 10-minute morning writing session and spend this time writing down triggers instead. Some triggers are quite obvious as they are embedded in repeated patterns or events from the Chapter 5 writing activity. I'd still encourage you to work through the following sections of this chapter. They contain a smorgasbord of ideas that may be helpful in spotting triggers (especially non-obvious ones).

We'll start by listing external triggers. External triggers are things that happen outside our body and are readily identified because we can see them and point to them in space. They include:

- lifting boxes of equipment off the floor

- kids climbing on your back

- standing up for long periods of time

- dinner with the in-laws

- assignments and exams

- sitting in an office chair

- sleeping on the wrong mattress

- *cold weather*

- *hot weather*

- *typing on a computer*

- *waking up and getting out of bed*

- *your boss berating you*

- *carrying groceries.*

This is a time and place to go with your gut feeling. Even if you are not sure, put it down just in case. Does bending your knee while walking upstairs cause pain? Or what about having to sit for long periods at work in an uncomfortable chair? These are both external triggers and have their genesis outside the body. It can be daunting at first because everything feels like a trigger. However, this isn't necessarily a bad place to start because it gives you a lot of material to work on.

Another approach could be to ask friends and family, "Hey, do you notice if I seem in pain when X happens?" Obviously, this approach depends on your social comfort level or openness, but external insight has led others down the path of fruitful writing sessions.

Do you still feel stuck and unsure if something is a trigger? One way you can move forward is by "backing up" in time or space from the trigger. Interrogate what happened immediately before the trigger. Could something else be the root cause?

Taking a step back in time from our trigger can provide us with valuable distance to make observations. When we "back up" from our triggers, we often encounter more existential "why" questions. This leads us down the path of triggers that are internal to our body or occur in our mind. We'll explore these internal triggers further in the next section.

When you have a draft list, revisit it and rank the more significant triggers at the top and work your way down. For example, something that happens many times per day (with no escape) or items that cause major pain sensations should be placed at the top. Less frequent or significant triggers can be shifted toward the bottom. The same goes for triggers that you may be unsure of. It's hard at first to sort the wheat from the chaff, but this is normal. With practice, observation, and refinement, you'll discover that this list largely centers on a handful of triggers.

To summarize the steps you need to take:

1. List triggers in your outside environment first.
2. Observe other triggers from times you were aware of your pain. (Use data points from your Chapter 5 writing activity.)
3. Reorder your list so the most critical triggers appear at the top.

Internal pain triggers can be challenging to find

Internal triggers are things that happen inside ourselves and can be more difficult to identify than triggers in the material world. We can't see, touch, or hear them (neither can our friends or family). They include:

- setting impossibly high standards for yourself (perfectionism)

- fear of turning our neck the wrong way

- putting pressure on ourselves to help other people

- feeling burdened with household chores

- not feeling good enough

- negative anticipation of work tomorrow

- worrying about the news media cycle.

Triggers that exist in our interior world are very hard to spot because we can't easily compare our mental thoughts to others as we would with physical actions. Consider the process of learning a new sport like golf. Sure, our swing won't be perfect on the first go, but we can improve by watching an instructor or coach—and even letting them physically adjust our grip or shoulder position until it is just right. To correct our technique, we can easily look at our golf instructor's swing, which has been crafted over 20 years of experience, and model the exact posture, body position, speed, and follow-through ourselves. It's easy to see our own deficiencies when compared with an expert golfer. This becomes much more difficult when we turn our minds inward.

To find internal triggers, we need to revisit the notes you took during your writing exercises. Was there a particular road your feelings or thought patterns took you down? There is often one or two that are front-of-mind and clearly in our consciousness.

The next step in identifying internal triggers involves stepping back from the external trigger. For instance, if twisting your back while at work causes serious pain but play-wrestling with your kids at home doesn't, that is a good suggestion of neuroplastic pain and that there might be an emotional connection at work. If the pain changes like this, we are already on the right track. Therefore, if your back hurts during work duties, understanding this trigger involves retracing the situation step by step. Is it because you get lumped with extra work? Is it because no one on your team offers help? Is it because you find it mentally hard to say no to superiors—and you feel guilty?

If the above two points did not produce sufficient fruit, just keep rewinding back from your pain. Ask yourself about your emotional state before you experienced pain. Sure, it might be a physical task, but lean in and ask "why." Asking "why" repeatedly, like a curious toddler, can help get to your core feelings and emotional drivers.

As we did above for external triggers, revise your draft list to rank the more intrusive ones and shift the less significant ones down toward the bottom end of your list.

By the end of this exercise, you'll be left with certain character traits or personality types. Examples could be fear, negative anticipation, goodism, perfectionism, and general busyness. These are big internal triggers (BITs) that seem to pervade everything. We will cover these individually in the following sections.

Follow these steps for listing internal triggers during your morning writing session:

1. List thoughts and feelings that keep appearing alongside pain (tease them out from your writing in Chapter 5).
2. Keep rewinding from an external trigger or pain flare-up and ask, "Why?" Why are you specifically aware of your pain now? What emotional state are you in?
3. Reorder your list so the most critical triggers appear at the top.

Before we move on, it's worth mentioning that the goal of finding triggers isn't to latch onto them and obsessively track them in minute detail. Please don't blame yourself when a trigger happens throughout the day, like becoming frustrated or not sleeping properly. This is just a draft list, so hold onto these triggers loosely.

Big internal triggers (BITs)

BIT 1: Fear is a predominant emotion with chronic pain

We react to uncomfortable sensations in one of two ways.

The first reaction is a healthy response to pain. Say we have been standing up and running around at work all day and are aware that our legs are a bit sore. We notice the discomfort and maybe take some corrective action, like sitting down, but it's no real problem. These kinds of pain experiences come and go within the space of just a few moments.

Further still, we do not fear this kind of discomfort prior to its occurrence. We think, "Whoops, that was a bit silly standing up all day at work without a break," rather than, "I cannot go to work today because I'm scared I will have to stand up and my legs will be killing me." The best thing about this first response is that we don't think twice about it. It happens to us a million times a day. We adjust in our seats if our muscles get a little stiff, we fix food to eat when we are hungry, and we get a glass of water after an exercise session. It's really not an issue. We don't fear it. We feel safe. We cut ourselves a lot of slack. We're quick to forgive our bodies because we go easy on ourselves. How we talk to ourselves is huge.

The second reaction is the one we are all too familiar with. This is led by fear. We fear the pain sensation before it happens or try to avoid it, not confront it. We even fear the thought of fearing the trigger in the first place. If we fall victim to the trigger, we have no sympathy for ourselves. Our internal monologue fires up: "I knew I shouldn't have pushed myself with the shopping. I'm so stupid."

Whereas in the first case our discomfort left soon after it arrived, this second pain path stays with us for the long run. We complain to our friends and family about this pain, creating an extra layer of social proof. Ultimately, this results in some form of mental or physical modification of our behavior, feeding the neuroplastic pain cycle.

Here are some points to review to address the internal fear trigger:

- Ask: Am I struck with pain or struck with fear? How would my life be better if I didn't have to fear pain?
- Review tangible evidence of a time when you were not in pain (Chapter 5). Can you relate them to your current situation?
- Review your pain levels on a given pain scale. Do they fit with your expectations?
- Explore, in ways that feel safe to you, challenging situations that may trigger your pain. The aim is to get insight and resolution to reduce fear (more in Chapter 7).

BIT 2: Replace negative anticipation with self-compassion

When bad things happen to us once, we expect them to happen again. This forms the basis of our second Big Internal Trigger (BIT): anticipation.

You can't anticipate acute pain because it happens suddenly and unexpectedly. You can and will anticipate neuroplastic pain before you have engaged in whatever activity causes it to flare up. Past experience shapes your future worries, but we can diminish negative anticipation by replacing it with self-compassion.

Anticipation is making a judgment about a hypothetical future situation before we have evidence to confirm or refute our hastily made conclusion. Anticipation can be positive or negative and plays a role in virtually every aspect of life, from hunger (anticipating dinner after a hard day of work) to drinking (that first glass of wine after a week at work) and social and romantic life (seeing friends, that first date, or other intimate relationships).

Do you anticipate pain sensations? For some, the mental torment and anguish with anticipation are worse than the pain itself. Take, for example, traveling with irritable bowel syndrome (IBS). You think about it in the weeks and days leading up to your holidays: Will there be bathrooms? I'll be really sick. I won't be able to do many day trips. Will I have to cancel? These multiple weeks of preceding anxieties and anticipation could be worse than suffering an actual week of physical IBS symptoms.

If you do, in fact, suffer a week of mild IBS on holidays, the cycle is concluded when rumination kicks in. It's like the polar opposite of anticipating a future event, dwelling on a past event. You start the cacophony of thoughts: Is it going to happen again? I'll never get better. Am I destined for a life of this? This anticipation-pain-rumination process repeats for future events.

Practice replacing anticipation with self-compassion:

1. We'll start at the end of a pain cycle: rumination. Try acknowledging you are ruminating; for example, "I've noticed that I'm dwelling on my pain now," and practice bringing it to a close. This is easier said than done, so distraction or self-care activities can help. Think: What can I do to stop feeding it now? How can I reduce the burden on myself?
2. Notice when you start to anticipate a chronic pain flare-up: "I'm worried that my pain will be bad tomorrow." From a lens of self-compassion, review evidence of your writing when previous episodes of pain have come and gone. Know that it will pass, and it may not be as terrible as you fear.

BIT 3: Goodism throws gasoline on internal triggers

The internal compulsion to please others and be a good person is called "goodism." It's damaging because it puts our own needs in a distant second place. This personality trait is regularly listed by experts as being a perpetuating factor of ongoing pain or psychosomatic illness.

Goodism is the philosophy that I must sacrifice my energy or needs for the exclusive benefit of others and then feel guilty about not giving more. Goodism causes your day-to-day encounters to rack up a huge debt of internal torment. No amount of patience and willpower can fix this, either. This can look like practicing patience with people pushing in line, someone cutting you off in traffic, demands from colleagues, or the compulsive need to respond to requests in the affirmative. It triggers pain because you can't say "no" or take agency for your own state. It's the opposite of empowerment.

Self-proclaimed goodists often admit that it causes them much resentment, leading to frustration toward the very people they love. This internal rage and anger are major causes of chronic pain.

You don't need to feel that you have to be your best self all the time. Achieve this by saying "no" to things, being intentional with your time, and not falling into the goodism trap. Goodism may not have started your pain, but it sure won't help you end it.

Learning to set boundaries is a fun experiment you get to play and is a sign your recovery is moving forward. Erode goodism by:

- Saying "no" to requests. You might still feel guilty; it might be difficult at first, but you should try to say "no" politely and firmly. Say "no" without hedging words, qualifications, or apologizing—you don't always have to give a reason.
- Or, invert the question. How will saying "yes" to this request aid my recovery?
- Put yourself first and ignore the next ask, email, phone call, notification, or event.
- People keep talking about finding "balance" in your work, social, family, and personal life. What happens if you drop some of the balls you are juggling? Explore what having a healthy balance means for you.

BIT 4: Perfectionism, control, and high expectations

When it comes to the sheer pervasiveness of internal triggers, nothing beats perfectionism. Perfectionism, by nature, breeds fear, anxiety, and hypothetical "what ifs." What if we aren't good enough? What if I fail at my job? What if I look stupid in front of that client?

Like goodism, it is often reported that people who suffer from neuroplastic pain suffer from high expectations and perfectionism. Reducing our perfectionistic tendencies and expectations can reduce what triggers our pain.

This internal trigger is unique in that we extend it beyond ourselves and onto our friends, family, and anonymous members of society. Friends can forget things —such as our birthday—on the odd occasion. Family may make choices that we don't always agree with. Society can be rude, illogical, and downright evil at times. It's all part of being human, something that we deny as perfectionists. When we see things that are "not as they should be," we create an environment for pain.

The result of the unrelenting high standard of perfection is control—controlling the above behaviors of ourselves, friends, family, and society. It is impossible to control others. By extension, is it impossible to truly control ourselves? We have all sorts of impulses and cravings.

Perfectionism ignores the humanity of weak, frail bodies and minds. Minds that naturally slip up and forget things from time to time. Bodies that get tired and have limits as to how much work they can do. A perfectionist who would settle for no less than a zero-out-of-ten—a bullseye. This runs counter to our goal of pain management: reducing pain to a three-out-of-ten level. We need to give up perfectionism to treat pain. We will always have discomforts and irritations.

Be on the lookout for perfectionist traits that trigger chronic pain:

An all-or-nothing approach to work, social life, and relationships. *If I can't do a 110% job, I'm a failure.*

Fix: Replace it with a "good enough" effort or an 80% complete job. Be open to what happens.

If it can't be perfect, it's not worth trying. This causes procrastination, avoidance, and doubt.

Fix: See procrastination as a consequence of perfectionism. Get started with smaller, less consequential tasks (aka quick wins).

Being hard on yourself and leaving no room for mistakes.

Fix: Be on the lookout for "should" statements. I "should" have pushed harder in that deal. I "should" have finished all the housework today. I "should" have spent more time with that friend.

Busyness. Busyness can be a symptom of perfectionism.

Fix: Write a to-do list with every single thing you need to do. Once you've written it, make a plan for eliminating some of these tasks. What can you delegate to someone else? What isn't completely necessary?

The goal of dealing with the trigger of perfectionism is being able to sit with the mess of life and realize that we can't always do a flawless job. Let some of the balls you've been juggling drop and roll away on the floor. Do a half-assed job from time to time. Reducing this mental burden goes a long way to minimizing pain.

Start validating or invalidating your list of pain triggers

You have a big list of triggers that might just aggravate your pain. This list is very helpful, but what is more important is the substantial change in mindset that trigger identification enables. We've gone from: "Ouch! It hurts. I need to make it stop!" to "Ouch! It hurts. *I wonder what triggers led to this pain?*" There is a subtle difference. One sentence ends with an exclamation point, the other with a question mark. Mindset changes like this are strong evidence of progress.

Speaking of progress, this section marks a milestone where we transition from observing our pain and writing about it to actively trying to stop or reduce the impact of triggers. This approach aims to reduce pain sensations as we continue the journey toward a three out of ten on the pain scale.

This list of triggers is nothing more than a list of assumptions; things that may or may not impact your pain. We might have a strong hunch or preconceived idea, but proving or disproving your assumptions with evidence is the main work in chronic pain management. A positive or negative result is still progress. If it was proven incorrect, and the item does not, in fact, cause pain—rejoice! This means you can cross it off your list and carry on living your life without worrying that this will be an issue. If it is a trigger, that's also good news because we can address it with proven methods in both the next section and Chapter 7.

The way you will validate triggers is by formulating a hypothesis statement. This gives you some distance between yourself and the trigger. You get to experiment with it and put it through its paces. The task at hand is not stopping the trigger but rather validating or invalidating it. This is very different from classical success or failure and win or lose. It's not a zero-sum game; it's just a process to work through.

A hypothesis involves a variable (the trigger) and some type of consequence or result (pain). A hypothesis can be structured in an "If... Then..." statement. Here are some examples to get you started:

Sample trigger hypotheses:

- *If I sit in my chair for a long time, then back pain will appear at a level of seven out of ten.*

- *If I move my neck to look over my shoulder, I will experience pain.*

- *If I think about work after hours, I will experience pain sensations greater than three out of ten.*

- *If I type at my office keyboard, then pain will happen in my arms.*

- *If I squat down to pick up something on the ground, then my knees will give way.*

- *When I wake up in the morning, my forehead will ache.*

- *When I am away from my workplace, doing a leisure activity, or on holidays, the pain will reduce in intensity.*

- *If I kick a football with friends, my back pain will temporarily become less severe.*

You'll observe that the last two statements are counter-examples. Flipping a proposition on its head can be a helpful breakthrough or build evidence for times when you are not in pain.

The hypothesis can be validated (proven correct) or invalidated (proven false). Statements, on the other hand, can't always be proven or disproven. They usually presuppose a given result "always happens" and include a lot of emotive language like "fear" or "killing me." Here are some erroneous comparisons to the above hypotheses.

Not a hypothesis:

- That chair makes my body feel sore. It always happens.
- My neck is in pain all the time; it just won't stop.
- My job causes this pain to happen.
- Arm pain happens all the time while typing.
- These kids are killing me when they leave their toys on the ground.
- I'm afraid of going to sleep because when I wake up, my headache will still be there.
- Work is a drag; I need it to be over.
- Pain has ruined me; I'll never be able to play sports again.

Finding the right words to say when talking about triggers and building hypotheses is a new skill. Few people have this ability without some degree of practice, patience, and repetition. Yes, identifying your own emotions and triggers can be practiced and refined with diligent and concerted effort.

A final word of warning: Do not form hypotheses during a major pain event or a trigger flare-up. It's hard to take a step back and think objectively when things are hot. Instead, use the 10-minute morning time slot to form a hypothesis and make observations to validate/invalidate it. Consider this a natural migration from the writing in Chapter 5.

Eliminate, redesign, or replace triggers (in that order)

Here's what you have achieved so far:

1. You've done a heap of writing.
2. You've found a bunch of triggers.
3. You've validated or invalidated them.

Now, what do you do with the validated ones?

The goal is to stop triggers from resulting in pain. Or at the first step, reducing the pain magnitude of a trigger. Note that I have not said to stop all the triggers because some simply can't be ceased. There is a difference between stopping the trigger and stopping the pain. The former is a cause, while the latter is a result.

In the hierarchy of control, elimination is ideal—just remove the trigger altogether. If that is not possible, we can move on to redesigning our environment or situation to mitigate against the trigger. Finally, we can consider replacing the problematic trigger with something else. Elimination, redesigning, and replacing all have their pros and cons and are highly situational. Let's check them out now.

The first thing to ask is, can we just eliminate the trigger? This can be an extreme step like moving to another country, changing jobs, or leaving a bad relationship. For someone whose pain is exacerbated by the cold weather, elimination could be moving from a cold sub-arctic environment to a sunny tropical country. Quitting a bad job may be a necessary move, too. For some, this might mean leaving a bad relationship or saying goodbye to a controlling friend. Elimination is much easier for external triggers because we can get real physical distance from them.

The potential side effect of elimination centers around unhelpful avoidance behaviors. Elimination may not give immediate closure or it may leave unresolved feelings at play (hello, internal triggers). Start small with quick wins that have little risk of negative consequences and are readily reversible. But if these side effects are a risk for you, engineering your environment may be a better option to reduce the trigger.

Redesigning, reconfiguring, or shaping your environment could mean setting personal and professional boundaries. At work, where interruptions all day long could trigger backache, this could mean talking with your boss to request tasks to be delivered via email. You can then engineer your day around checking email, say, once between 11:30 AM and 12:00 PM. At home, this could mean an agreement with a partner not to raise worrisome issues after 8:00 PM, or better still, redesign your environment to quarantine "worry time." Structuring some additional time off, away from your triggers, during the week can work wonders—like taking a walk in a nearby park.

When we redesign our environment to accommodate neuroplastic symptoms, we may unintentionally reinforce those symptoms by catering to them excessively. For example, using a non-medically necessary knee brace or using the idea of "redesigning" as an excuse *not* to do physical exercise can actually hinder progress toward your goals and managing pain effectively. While these adjustments may provide temporary relief, they may ultimately perpetuate the cycle of pain by neglecting to address the underlying emotional causes.

It's essential to pause and reflect on your motives behind these actions. A good question to ask yourself is, "Am I treating the underlying emotion-driven neuroplastic cause, or am I trying to fix the physical symptoms?" This question prompts us to consider whether our actions are truly addressing the root issue or merely masking the surface symptoms.

The last step is a substitution of one trigger for another. It could be delegating a task to someone else, thereby replacing the external task trigger with the need to engage someone else. For instance, engaging a gardener or cleaner if house chores cause pain (though I realize for many of us, myself included, this is a luxury that cannot be easily afforded). The main side effect of substitution is enabling habits that may run counter to your goals—like eliminating grocery shopping and meal preparation by delegating to a fast-food restaurant.

Get closure by focusing on one trigger at a time

Eliminating, redesigning, or substituting every trigger at once is a surefire way to make you feel overwhelmed and burnt out. This will ultimately ensure that nothing changes in the long run. Like everything in pain management, the "secret" is little steps, taken consistently, in the direction toward the final objective. Remember that the final objective isn't necessarily to eliminate the trigger but rather reduce the resulting pain that it causes.

In practice, this means working on one trigger at a time. You have full permission to ignore the others until you've wrapped this up and have reached closure. So, what on earth is closure? Closure is being able to look back and observe the trigger without the trigger staring back at you. It is being able to poke and prod it without it agitating you back. It is being able to automatically do the opposite of the symptoms it once gave you. It means you no longer fear the trigger or experience pain greater than three out of ten.

External help may be needed, such as working with your doctor or psychologist to enable techniques to reduce the impact of triggers. The benefit of working with a professional is learning techniques that can be applied across the spectrum of your trigger list. Once you have crossed off the first trigger, tackle the second one. It will fall quicker than the first but slower than the third.

Use somatic tracking on triggers you can't seem to budge

This chapter aimed to cover two things: 1) identifying what causes pain flare-ups by giving you awareness and knowledge of triggers, and 2) enabling a mindset change to give you space from your triggers by either eliminating, redesigning, or replacing them.

A measure of success is when you have a pain sensation, pause, take five minutes, and think about what triggered your pain this time and how you might creatively engineer that trigger out of your daily life.

But we've tiptoed around the most pressing question: What happens if a trigger just can't be changed? It could be your family, your mortgage, that pervasive sense of perfectionism, or deep, long-held insecurities. What happens when we can't just engineer them out of our lives like we would cross off items on a grocery list?

Back in Chapter 3 we saw that chronic pain sufferers have faced this very problem before. The peer-reviewed research tells us that somatic tracking is the best solution for drastically reducing pain. This means we can now focus our efforts on our final activity: somatic tracking.

Your takeaways from Chapter 6

A pain flare-up can be rethought of as a trigger flare-up. A trigger is an automatic cue that makes you aware of pain sensations in your body.

A trigger can be:

- External to your body, such as sitting in a chair, typing at a keyboard, or twisting your neck at work.
- Internal and feelings-based, including perfectionism, insecurities, or resentment about something.

Your daily 10-minute writing session will now shift to identifying triggers. When you have a list of 10 items, you can validate or invalidate them. Use an "If... Then..." hypothesis statement: "If I sit in my chair for a long time, then back pain will appear at a level of seven out of ten."

Finally, see if you can alleviate the pain caused by the trigger by:

- Eliminating it—like quitting a high-pressure, stressful job.
- Reconfiguring it—setting boundaries for your time.
- Replacing it—delegating the trigger-causing task to someone else.

7. Somatic tracking is the high-impact method of treating neuroplastic pain

This chapter will close the loop on the active steps of our pain management system. We've explored the benefits of emotional expression through writing and how this helps us spot and then eliminate things that trigger pain. But pain is a complex experience that cannot always be "written away" with the stroke of a pen. Therefore, the last tool in our arsenal for reducing pain is somatic tracking. You may have heard about somatic tracking as one of the components of Pain Reprocessing Therapy.[*] At a high level, somatic tracking invites you to tune into a sensation that you interpret as pain, or as anticipatory to pain, and observe and connect with it.

Tracking is all about following behind something, inquiring, and investigating with curiosity. The opposite of

---

[*] You can learn more background about Pain Reprocessing Therapy in *The Way Out: A Revolutionary, Scientifically Proven Approach to Healing Chronic Pain* by Alan Gordon and Alon Ziv.

tracking is jumping in front to direct it or control it to do your bidding. Like following behind an animal from a safe distance, somatic tracking teaches us to observe our bodily (soma) sensations, without trying to change them, from a position of safety and self-compassion. It's a psychological intervention that changes how we make sense of the world around us and inside of us. With practice, this deactivates pain.

Research is clear that this method has a high probability of success in treating neuroplastic pain. Following this approach gives us the upper hand with pain recovery because it means we'll make the most of our time and energy. If there is only one thing to do to weaken pain sensations, this is it.

This new chapter signifies a change in your morning 10-minute session as you transition from "identifying triggers" to "somatic tracking." Here's how you will become more adept in somatic tracking as you journey from total beginner to pretty-darn-good practitioner:

1. As with anything new, we start by ensuring somatic tracking fits with our big goal of pain management.
2. Learn about the benefits and potential barriers that we may come across before they happen so you don't get demotivated and give up.
3. Equip yourself with the vocabulary (tools) to practice somatic tracking.

4. Practice the somatic tracking process by starting simply. We'll focus on your breathing because it's a simple sensation that happens thousands of times per day.
5. Grow your somatic tracking skills by achieving a full body scan of pain sensations.

We'll end with troubleshooting some common problems. As with the previous sections, I recommend reading the whole chapter first to see the entire journey and then selectively revisiting it to practice the exercises.

Deactivate pain by decoupling your emotions from your bodily sensations

It's notoriously challenging to articulate the goal of psychological intervention because no one can show you a "before and after" photo as we would with dramatic weight loss or a spectacular house renovation. So, before we start somatic tracking, let's check in to see how it aligns with our management goal.

In Chapter 2, we targeted reducing our pain level to three or less on a 0–10 scale. The reasoning is that a pain level below three out of ten is a phenomenon that "I can ignore most of the time" or "I am aware of it only when I pay attention to it." Somatic tracking aligns with our big goal of reducing pain sensations because it stops you from being aware of, responding to, and being influenced by your pain.

We achieve this goal by deliberately shifting our minds toward what our body *feels* instead of what our brain *thinks*. Compare the two statements: "There is a throbbing discomfort in my lower back," versus, "My back is in terrible pain that won't stop." You can feel a "discomfort" in your *body*, but you *think* it is a "terrible pain that won't stop." The "thinking" part is a reaction, judgment, and rumination, and our aim is to become aware of this mental process as it occurs.

Ultimately, this line of thinking can lead to pain catastrophizing, which can cause you to feel more intense pain. It's a vicious cycle. The first step for unwinding this is by feeling your pain instead of thinking about your pain. Here's how we can spot the difference.

Feeling your pain (good progress):

- There is a numb feeling in my wrists.
- My neck has a sharp sensation.
- There is a dull ache in my back that seems to move around.

Thinking about your pain (less ideal):

- My pain has been going on for five whole years.
- This is excruciating, and I can't go on.
- My back pain feels like I am being stabbed all day. It is impossible to ignore.
- I can never twist my back again.

This habit is hard to break, but you can create a new habit to think of pain as benign, not threatening, or just a fleeting sensation. As you continue with somatic tracking, you will get significantly better at not reacting to and ruminating on the sensations of pain and discomfort. With practice, you will become an expert at accepting that your brain does things beyond your control, understanding that you can't always dictate its course, and preventing yourself from falling headfirst into a rumination spiral.

With any undertaking, there are caveats. The caveat here is that there will always be discomforts in life. Your neck is going to feel stiff in the morning, just like everyone else. Your knees may twinge when you bend over to pick up a toy off the floor, just like everyone else. Your back is still going to ache after standing during a long work shift, just like everyone else. It is not realistic for anyone of any age, health status, or ability to eliminate these bodily nuisances.

So, what do "normal" people do when they notice a momentary hit of pain? They just brush it aside. They don't catastrophize or ruminate. And somatic tracking can enable us to do just that.

Redefine "pain" as a "sensation"

During the somatic tracking exercises, we will make a very deliberate change in language around pain. Instead of using the word "pain" explicitly, I invite you to use the word "sensation" or "signal." I would also encourage you to play with the idea of this sensation being "temporary." It's not a permanent, irreversible thing but rather something that ebbs and flows. This allows us to approach neuroplastic pain from a more neutral and objective angle. After all, pain is just a sensation.

If the jump of redescribing "pain" as a "temporary sensation" is too big of an initial step, I would invite you to play with an intermediate description instead. Terms like a "painful sensation" or a "temporary painful signal" might help make the transition easier. This is something you will have to practice and repeat before it feels more at home. "Sensations" can be seen as temporary, whereas "pain" is often interpreted as more persistent and destructive.

With this newfound definition, it's worth flagging that negative emotions and feelings themselves aren't bad or something we need to battle against. We are turning toward negative emotions, and this helps us tune into them. Tuning in empowers us to resolve emotions rather than keep them stuck in our bodies. Negative emotions are still powerful, but we have learned how to give them space and interrogate them from a distance.

Somatic tracking is challenging because it's counterintuitive

Somatic tracking has enormous benefits for chronic pain relief, but that doesn't mean it's easy or without its challenges. It does mean that we need to have a plan for when we do face obstacles. It's good to know this before the fact so you can approach it sober-mindedly instead of being surprised by barriers if or when they appear. Here is a quick overview of the benefits and challenges.

Benefits of somatic tracking include:

- Scientifically validated: Somatic tracking has been scientifically validated as an effective method for reducing neuroplastic pain to lower than three out of ten. This has been backed up with fMRI scans that show the function of a chronic pain-riddled brain before and after treatment.
- Control and privacy: You're in the driver's seat and can practice as much as you like in the privacy of your own space.
- Safety: Somatic tracking is a safe approach to pain management as it does not involve surgery or carry any medical side effects.
- Cost free: There are no associated costs involved, making it accessible to all individuals regardless of financial circumstances.
- Flexibility: You can stop at any point with no consequences or withdrawal side effects.
- Non-medicated: Somatic tracking is a non-medicated approach and does not negatively interact with any medication you may be taking.

There are some challenges we'll need to overcome. The good news is that you can apply these fixes during your daily practice to instantly level up.

CHALLENGE 1: At the most basic level, we need the right **descriptor words for pain sensations** (adjectives). Describing the attributes or quality of chronic pain requires the right toolset. Adjectives give important details to make the most of the time you spend on somatic tracking.

FIX 1: Use the glossary in the following section, "Better adjectives are the tool for more effective sensation tracking," to upskill.

CHALLENGE 2: If you're anything like me, it can be **counterintuitive**. This is a big one. Deliberately exposing yourself to the thing you have avoided for so long is undeniably a barrier because it just doesn't *feel* right. You have become skilled at fleeing from pain, not interrogating it in a safe manner. It requires a mindset change from "I know that my pain is killing me" to "I wonder what this feeling is?"

FIX 2: We'll start by practicing with something that is not our pain in this chapter (see *Start with this warm-up exercise: feeling your breath for five minutes*).

CHALLENGE 3: Following on from the point above, it takes a lot of **vulnerability**. By vulnerable, I mean you are exposed to something that has the ability (or imagined potential) to cause harm and pain. It's another mindset change. We are vulnerable when we tell a close friend about our failing romantic relationship—for a split second, the power is in our friend's hands to either do good or harm. We are vulnerable when we make a stand for our point of view or opinion at work—for a moment, our whole career can hinge on the reaction of our boss. It's no longer in our control, but somebody else's.

FIX 3: When we are vulnerable it rarely turns out as bad as we imagined. Often, we are left with a deep sense of relief, achievement, and growth.

CHALLENGE 4: It is a skill that you will probably fail at first. The first time you perform a new skill, you will likely suck at it, like everyone else.

FIX 4: We will map the progress and steps throughout the somatic tracking activities to set you up for success, even if it feels like you are not getting anywhere initially.

CHALLENGE 5: It is hard to **maintain long term**. This is a consequence of "cost free," "flexibility," and "non-medicated" in the benefits list above. It's hard to maintain because you can just stop at any point without consequences. There is no doctor chasing you for appointments and time commitments, no money on the line, and no nasty side effects from quitting cold turkey.

FIX 5: We will use time in our established morning writing routine. We will talk about this and other roadblocks toward the end of this chapter (see *Overcoming common roadblocks for somatic tracking*).

Now that we are clear on the approach, benefits, and potential roadblocks, we can start working on the tools and processes to make somatic tracking successful in the long term.

Better adjectives are the tool for more effective sensation tracking

Somatic tracking requires two things—the first being "tools and techniques" and the other being the "process." Just like a hammer, chisel, and saw are tools, the process is the manual carpentry work to build your new cabinet. A process is a method that brings the basic tools and raw inputs together, transforming them.

Before we enter the carpentry shop of somatic tracking, you need a few tools. The first one is the tool to accurately describe your sensation. This means expanding our vocabulary beyond "it hurts." It's very important to name the sensation accurately as you monitor it throughout your body. This may sound condescending or dismissive, but the unavoidable fact is that you must get better at describing your pain to a high degree of specificity. Finding the right adjective helps to describe it and remove unknowns.

The good news is that thinking about adjectives means you are shifting your mindset to be more open and curious. Naming your pain as a specific sensation helps you track it. Does it feel like a burning first thing in the morning? Does it manifest as a dull ache during periods of major stress? Is it closer to a tingling numbness compared to an acute stabbing? Neuroplastic pain is known to shift and change in quality like this.

Here is the toolset for describing sensations:

Acute, sharp, or stabbing. Like tissue being sliced apart. Usually felt on the outer surface of the body part in question.

Burning. A sharp pain close to the skin. There is a distinct feeling of heat, like a sunburn or touching a hot pan. You may get a similar feeling from eating chili or wasabi.

Dull or aching. Usually felt deeper than the skin. Hard to place exactly because it can be vague. If it is in your back and you can't locate it at first, be methodical. Start at the top of your head and move down to your bottom. Where was the pain?

Numb or tingling. Like pins and needles. Similar to the feeling of lying on a body part and feeling numb due to loss of circulation. Next time you sit or lie in an awkward position that causes pins and needles, use this as an excellent opportunity to soak it in.

Throbbing. What else throbs? Is this your heart-beat? Start by finding your heart. Use your hands and fingers to physically locate it. Feel the peak of each pulse and notice the space in between.

Itching or scratching. This is what happens when you have a stray hair that is scratching your neck or a stick that brushes against your leg. You may get a similar feeling with eczema or an old scab.

Tension or tightness. This is like the sensation you get from clenching your fist or jaw for a long time. An example could be how focusing intently on a task causes your forehead or neck to tense.

Stiffness, discomfort, restlessness. The perfectly normal result of sitting in an office chair or driver's seat for several hours or when we first wake up and our body feels inflexible.

The point of learning these adjectives is that if the only tool we have is a hammer, we will see every problem as a nail. If we describe every occurrence of minor discomfort as "killing me," we risk incorrectly mischaracterizing sensations and ending in less-effective somatic tracking. How else are we to describe the sensation of the muscle tension of sitting in a chair for three hours if the only descriptor we have is a "sharp stabbing?" Exploring these sensations gives you more tools for highly productive somatic tracking.

Start with this warm-up exercise: feel your breath for five minutes

To date, we've made progress in understanding our goal and getting new tools for describing pain. But this has been theoretical knowledge. Therefore, it's time to change gears into "experiential learning mode" so we can learn by doing.

The focus now is on cultivating awareness of your breath, and this section achieves its goal if you've dedicated five minutes to practicing this mindfulness exercise. You might wonder why we're beginning with breathing rather than immediately addressing your chronic pain. There are two reasons for this.

The first reason is that intentionally observing and sensing our pain can be uncomfortable, to say the least. If we fear it, we may avoid it altogether, leaving the somatic tracking process stranded. Starting with a sensation that is not our pain helps overcome this potential barrier later.

Secondly, breathing is one of the few bodily systems that are under both conscious and unconscious control. We can intentionally think about and shape our breathing—like taking a deep breath in before we dive underwater and exhaling only when we resurface, and not a moment sooner. But if we stop thinking about breathing, it doesn't matter. The body kicks in and puts it on autopilot. Compare breathing to, say, digestion in our stomach. We can't control digestion and hence don't give it a second thought because it's completely unconscious.

Consciously focusing on a bodily function, like breathing, shapes the unconscious behavior of our body. Deep breathing calms the nervous system, which is stuck on high alert with neuroplastic pain. Breathing tells our brains that we are safe and not in danger. It's a unique peephole into our unconscious world that our body gives us. For a brief moment, we get to reach in, adjust some gears, set things in motion, and shut the hood.

I'll now invite you to practice somatic tracking during your morning sessions. Let's start with the following.*

Morning somatic exercise

This will take five minutes of active time, plus a minute or two beforehand to set your phone alarm.

Most people are comfortable doing this sitting down on something soft like a sofa. During the five minutes, close your eyes and notice when you breathe in, and then observe when you breathe out. Notice your chest as it fills with air and how your stomach moves as it is released.

---

* Many of you have commented that you prefer to listen to these somatic exercises. I've recorded exercises from this chapter and made the audio freely available for you to access here: www.pastpainbook.com/audio

That's it. Just experience what happens during an inhale and exhale.

I bet you'll be lucky to last two seconds.

It's frustrating stuff, but we can learn from it. So, try again—without forcing it—to see how far you get. Ask yourself, "Was that a short breath or a long breath?" or "Does the breath feel the same or different?" A few seconds later, you'll be attacked by the thought of your neighbor's kid who kicks a soccer ball inside the apartment above you. It's impossible not to be distracted. Breathing exercises like this are about being aware of the distractions as much as focusing on the breath.

Move your attention back to breathing. Slowly work through your five senses. What can you hear during an inhale? What can you taste in your mouth? What do you smell as air rushes in through your nose? Close your eyes and mentally note what you feel. What do you feel in your stomach during an exhale?

And like that, the exercise will be over. Well done.

This exercise is all about noticing how fickle your brain is when trying to track a bodily sensation. Your breath is just an easy benchmark to measure your brain activity.

Anxious thoughts come and go. Uncomfortable sensations pop into your head. Bad memories flicker back and forth. The value is in exposing your brain for what it is and standing back and realizing that ideas seem to come and go at random. It's like a wayward puppy, excitedly running from person to person, scent to scent, or dog to dog. Sniffing momentarily and then moving on. Despite what you may think, it's largely out of your control.

Respond to distractions by:

1. Noticing a distraction has happened.
2. Refocusing back on your breath.
3. Scanning through your senses.

Practice this foundational skill daily for at least one week. As a rule of thumb, you're ready to move on to the next section if you can feel the way your breath changes as you monitor it over several minutes.

Get used to performing somatic tracking with a body scan

Basic somatic tracking is all about finding one bodily sensation and having it in our awareness. Once it is in our awareness, we can track it and follow how it feels within our body over time. This exercise is all about getting familiar with our bodily sensations more broadly to identify and then pinpoint one or two key sensations for more in-depth somatic tracking in the next section.

You'll need to give yourself permission to take 10 minutes to do this. Commit to practicing it for 10 minutes, no matter how distracted or uncertain you are.* This means you have set an actionable goal. You know the step you need to take (somatic tracking), the timeframe (10 minutes), and the location (at the breakfast table before coffee). Ideally, you want to tack this onto an existing habit (also known as habit stacking) to make sure it sticks.

Now that you've got a spare moment, the second pre-work huddle is a temporary change in mindset: be curious and open about bodily sensations. Curiosity is the ability to understand something without passing judgment on it. Curiosity is a skill, and it's centered on asking open questions instead of closed questions or statements. Things like "I wonder..." or "What if..." are excellent. Statements like "This hurts" or closed questions like "When will it stop?" are not conducive to curiosity.

Curiosity has the added benefit of enabling you to be in a safe and compassionate mindset. It's near impossible to engage in curiosity-type thinking when you're in the clutches of a fight or flight danger response. People with chronic pain rarely activate this curiosity mindset as they supposedly need to make life-or-death judgments, not sit and ponder something. Open-ended questions activate

---

* Some early readers of this book commented that "more is not more" when it comes to somatic tracking. Limiting somatic tracking time to 10 minutes is the sweet spot. Trying to do more than that can switch your brain "on" to trying to force something to happen, which is counterproductive.

these mental centers, steering away from immediate judgment and fostering self-compassion. Ultimately, this practice helps you relax.

Now that we have the time and mindset change, we'll start basic somatic tracking with a body scan.

This section aims to have awareness of the feelings inside your body from head to toe. That means you could say to a friend nearby, "My ears are ringing," "My stomach is on edge," "My calves feel a bit tight," or "I can feel the firm dining room chair under my butt." This is good; this is the aim.

Morning somatic exercise

Sit in a relaxed space and close your eyes. Practice noticing a few breaths to get you in the mood.

Start at your head. What do you feel in your head? How about your forehead? If your jaw is tense, release it. Breathe in and out slowly. Do you feel anything in your sinus behind your nose? How about the back of your scalp?

Move to your neck. Is it tight and constricted? Or active and alert? What does swallowing feel like? How about your shoulders? Are they slouched forward or back and tight?

Travel down your arms and into your wrists and fingers. Are they warm or cold? Clenched or hanging loosely? Are your arms or hands making contact with another part of your body?

Move back up your shoulders and down your back. This can be challenging for some, but just walk through it and see what happens. Start between your shoulders. Can you feel your spine and trace it down? All the way to your lower back and pelvis?

How about your hips? Do they feel tight and closed, or open and excited—as if you are about to play your favorite sport and you are in the zone called "flow?" Focus on the surface you are sitting on. What does this interface feel like? Try to remain neutral when observing, neither good nor bad. It just is.

Let's go further down your legs and to the very soles of your feet. What do your hamstrings and quadriceps feel like? Have you subconsciously tensed them as if they are ready for action, or are they relaxed and maybe cross-legged or draping across a lounge? Keep going further down to your knees, calves, and the extremity of your toes. What does it feel like to wiggle them?

Nearly there. Let's work back to your abdomen (the front of your back that we scanned before).

Can you focus on the depths of your stomach? If it was speaking to you, what would it say? Can you feel your diaphragm? Trace your esophagus and windpipe from your chest right up to your mouth and out into the atmosphere.

For the last step, we'll engage with our senses. What do you hear? What sounds are close by? What sounds are far away? What do you hear inside you?

Engage your tongue. What can you taste? Is it a recent meal or drink? Or just the gummy dryness of your mouth?

What can you smell? Starting from the furthest sphere away from you and working closer right up to your nose.

What sensations do you feel with your skin? The intent is to find external stimuli that interact with the outermost surface of your skin.

Softly open your eyes as if you are waking from a deep sleep. What do you see both far away and slowly drawing your sight close by? What color, pattern, or shape catches your eye?

Take a few more breaths before fully opening your eyes and completing this first session.

What should it feel like after completing it?

We've talked about quick wins, but this is a big one. Be satisfied and proud—you have done a major task and performed a technique that, with practice, reduces neuro-plastic pain. Don't feel guilty about feeling good about yourself or downplay your achievement. You set out to do something and achieved it. This is an immensely rewarding experience. It feels good to get better at something.

Just as with breathing, you likely have firsthand experience of how easily your brain can be distracted by other ideas or intrusive thoughts. If thoughts and distractions pop into your head readily, only to disappear just as soon, maybe some of the thoughts you have about your pain are just as fleeting and should receive little to no attention.

You should aim to develop better skills in identifying and naming sensations in a neutral, matter-of-fact way without rushing to classify them as good or bad. Achieving three significant accomplishments in 10 minutes is pretty good if you ask me.

It's unlikely there will be any big revelations or a light-bulb moment—if there is, great. Instead, revelations and growth come through many small repetitions. We're building a habit here. If you ever feel stuck or unsure what to do on your journey of building the somatic tracking habit, this is the section to return to and practice.

Advanced somatic tracking

With the work we've done to date, we haven't made any observations on our pain sensations. This has been deliberate. The main process of somatic tracking is all about noticing and describing the way our body functions and changes over time. And we've practiced this with breathing before moving on to a full body scan.

Now, it's time to zero in on the pain sensations. The goal is to focus on this sensation to describe it and see what it does over time. Finally, at the end of our 10 minutes, we'll check in to see how this body signal has changed, if at all.

Morning somatic exercise

Step one: Find where the sensation is and describe the location in detail. For example, if the sensation is coming from your knee, learn about it. Is it at the top, bottom, near the surface, or deep within? How does it compare to your other knee? Don't move on until you are formulating it in specific words: "The sensation is at the top surface of my right knee."

Describe the characteristics of the localized sensation from the adjectives listed previously. Is it tingly? Dull? Sharp?

Step two: Sit with the sensation. You don't need to do anything to it, you don't need to get rid of it, you don't need to change it, and you don't need to make it stop. Just notice it.

Staying still and embracing the sensation is hard because pain signals are designed for and effective at alerting us to do something. It is meant to make us respond and is the opposite of what somatic tracking does. It's like if we were meeting a friend for coffee, and they greeted us with, "Hello, it's wonderful to see you. How have you been?" What if we didn't reply and just held their gaze and watched their reaction out of curiosity? Maybe they might repeat the greeting, get uncomfortable, and wave in front of our faces. Eventually, they might walk away. It's a super awkward situation. We are doing this with the pain.

Step three: Follow the sensation for the next 10 minutes. Does it move? What does it feel like to sit with it? How often does your brain wander? What is it like to just feel it but do (and think) absolutely nothing? How has the quality of the sensation changed? Could you use a different adjective? Has the magnitude increased, decreased, or remained constant?

Step four: Finally, remind yourself that this sensation is neuroplastic—it's brain signals that have been learned by your brain, not damage to your body. Remind yourself of times or situations in the past when the sensation has temporarily reduced or weakened. Remind yourself that you are safe, and you are building a powerful and durable method of reducing neuroplastic pain.

Speaking positive phrases to yourself can be helpful here: "My back is *healthy*" instead of "My back is not *damaged*," or "I am *safe*" instead of "I am not in *danger*."

Well done on taking yet another step toward sustainable pain management. You have taught your brain a new way of dealing with pain.

Here is some evidence that you've made quick wins:

- You felt your target sensation for the first time intentionally and with curiosity.
- You feel that what is happening in your body is OK and likely to be benign.
- The sensation moves around.
- The quality changes.

If this all feels a bit too much, it's perfectly OK to back up and spend more time on breathing techniques or a body scan. As with anything, you'll need to practice somatic tracking to become more proficient. We're building a durable and effective neuroplastic pain management system with the aim of long-term sustainability.

Decouple pain from emotions by reappraising

Looping back to the start of the chapter, I mentioned that the big goal of somatic tracking is to decouple the painful sensation that you feel from the emotions and thoughts you think about. This is done through "reappraisal," and it concludes your somatic tracking work.

Reappraisal is one of those words that is rarely used in everyday conversation. It involves a re-evaluation process where you can essentially wipe the slate clean and bring in an expert to provide a new perspective. When I think of reappraising, I think of reappraising home values. You know how, after owning a place for 10 or 20 years, its value can change? Despite having a gut feeling about it, you call in an appraiser who offers an independent assessment. They cut through the decades of emotional attachment or connection with the neighborhood and provide a calm, measured, and objective opinion of the value of something.

Reappraisal is value based. The value of a home increased. The value of an artwork or an antique just skyrocketed—or maybe it dropped to zero after being assessed as a fake. This is what pain reappraisal is. It's changing how you value pain. Doing it yourself is often hard because we are so emotionally invested that we can overvalue certain aspects while undervaluing other features we might not have expertise in.

Discomfort, irritations, pain, and tightness are all normal sensations from a healthy body that require reappraising. Your task is to tell your body that they are safe. Here are the ways you can do it (and what to avoid):

- "They cannot hurt me." (I'm in permanent danger.)
- "This is a minor discomfort." (This is killing me.)
- "My body is healthy and strong." (There has to be something dangerously wrong.)
- "This feeling will pass soon." (This feeling is going to last forever.)
- "Thank you for bringing my attention to this tension. You don't need to warn me anymore." (I'm always in pain.)
- "It's a false alarm." (How bad is it now?)
- "I can be at ease." (I won't be able to work ever again.)
- "A-ha! This sensation was triggered by X." (Everything causes pain.)

Changing our values on something like pain is coupled with changing our belief about pain. Revisiting Chapter 4 may be a helpful reminder that neuroplastic pain can be treated.

Finally, reappraising does not mean *reattributing*. Reappraisal does not mean changing your mind by assuming that your back pain was once caused by stenosis but is now caused by tight lumbar muscles and a pinched nerve. This is not reappraising the present situation; it's trying to shift the believed cause. Are you changing the psychological value of your pain, or are you trying to change the physical cause?

Self-reattribution to another physical diagnosis runs the risk of embarking on another downward cycle of tests, scans, surgery, and general health anxiety. This can reinforce the idea that "there must be something wrong with my body" instead of the idea that "there must be something wrong with how my mind processes sensations."

The rest of this chapter is devoted to overcoming roadblocks and barriers on your way to establishing somatic tracking as a treatment method.

Your first few attempts are supposed to be a mess

Creating proficiency in a new skill invites a lot of room for mess. Did you ever succeed the first time you did something new? Probably not. I've recently been taking steps to improve my cooking skills, and it's been an exercise in patience. Even when I have a recipe right in front of me, all the food prepared, and the right equipment at hand, it just never seems to turn out perfect on the first go. I'm learning that perfection is not helpful and that aiming for "average" or "a little bit better than last time" is a better place to start. Somatic tracking is an experiential skill, and we need to learn by actually doing it without worrying it won't be perfect on the first few attempts. The point is to just make an attempt and try.

As you practice it, you will find a natural rhythm. Don't worry about following the script exactly, doing it "right" or "wrong." Just get the basic points. Start noticing what is going on in your body at the time. Don't try to change it. Don't judge it as bad, painful, sore, or achy. Finally, notice how darn hard it is to pay attention in a relaxed state. If your pain changes in sensation or quality or shifts around—good. That's a successful attempt.

Practice regularly, not haphazardly

Now that we know somatic tracking is one of the most effective ways of stopping chronic pain, the question is: When should I do it?

You may have heard lots of answers like:

- Just do it all the time!
- Only when you are in pain.
- Only when you are *not* in pain.
- Each tracking experience is unique to the individual and depends on your situation.

Did you spot the problem with the above answers? If you are given the option to do something at any time, you will do it none of the time. It feels abstract compared to the obligations and tasks I must do throughout the week. I need to do the grocery shopping before the kids come home from school. I need to keep my doctor's appointment at 9:15 AM. I am going to a friend's house for dinner at 6 PM and need to make something to share. These are all specific tasks—they have an aim, a time-frame, and an outcome. These tangible responsibilities are easy to keep and push out abstract tasks, like "doing somatic tracking."

The problem is that this takes insane amounts of willpower—something that neither you nor I have when times are good, let alone when things are bad. Worse still, if I don't have enough willpower, I am not motivated to try. Therefore, practice somatic tracking at a regular time and place so you don't have to rely on your memory, mood, or willpower.

If you find yourself stuck or not sure when to practice, maintain your morning sessions to grow in proficiency. Do it in a safe and comfortable position, like being seated or lying down. This notches up quick wins and builds momentum.

Pre-commit to doing somatic tracking when you experience a trigger

Safely experiencing pain is something that doesn't normally happen outside the confines of our 10-minute morning time. We normally experience pain in an unsafe environment. That could be a physical place, like a high-pressure office building, a social environment, like a nasty family situation, or a bad emotional headspace, like when we are feeling down and wound up with anxiety. Retreating into our safe place to practice tracking is excellent when we first learn somatic tracking skills. But I wonder if we can travel a little further outside our comfort zone to level up.

If you want to challenge yourself, try practicing somatic tracking at the time of day and in the environment where you typically experience pain. This often coincides with the task or bodily movement that triggers your pain. Your pain trigger has now become an opportunity for somatic tracking.

You can look through your list of triggers to make pre-commitments for when pain may arise. Before you bend your knees to lift a shopping bag from the ground, tell yourself, "I am going to do some somatic tracking during this movement." Or if you need to finish off some admin work at your computer and typing causes arm pain, tell yourself, "I will do some somatic tracking as soon as I start typing."

Practicing somatic tracking while in pain is effective because it is a "corrective experience." A corrective experience is when a bad trigger event happens* but with a

---

* If pain is agonizingly high, it is unlikely you will benefit from a corrective experience. You don't want to reinforce the faulty wiring in your brain by forcing yourself to "just push through it." If this is the case,

new, resolved ending. The key to somatic tracking is to feel the bodily pain and sensations—to say, "Bring it on. I'm ready to see what it feels like without trying to fix it." Instead of letting your emotions control your pain, resulting in anguish, you can face your trigger, knowing that the outcome will be "just another bodily sensation."

Being able to do somatic tracking while faced with pain symptoms is the pinnacle of pain management. It's not something that can be forced with willpower alone, but rather the natural culmination of the skills you have developed in writing about triggers, practicing noticing your breath, scanning your body, and reappraising "terrible pain" into "bodily sensations."

Overcoming common roadblocks for somatic tracking

Each time you practice somatic tracking, you dismantle the fortress of pain brick by brick. Eventually, there will be no bricks left. The key is to walk over, reach down, pick up a brick, and just start. But there are some common barriers or roadblocks that people face as they begin dismantling the first few bricks.

You still **fight the pain sensation** or want it to go away. Even if you know and believe 100% that it is neuro-

safety behaviors, distraction, and self-care is your best bet. Simply not making it worse is still a step in the right direction. Press pause on active pain management for now-.

plastic, you fight it with your emotions. Signs you are fighting it are if you catch yourself saying things like, "Argh! Make it stop," "I need to fix it," "Another flare-up has happened," and "Why isn't it getting better?" This is the main reason that people give up. In five minutes, they may have been able to change their factual beliefs about pain management, but the emotional response often lags by weeks or months.

Even if you know and say, "I'm OK" and "I know this isn't dangerous," emotions and facts are two very different sides of the coin. Factually knowing that bingeing on junk food is bad doesn't change the wonderful emotions we feel during a snaccident! An emotional response leads when we want something desirable and lags when we don't want to do something. In Chapter 2, we talked about how facts don't always change behaviors; instead, behaviors change behavior. Start by doing small behaviors until they shape your beliefs.

This leads us to the second point: **practicing**. Practicing helps change your emotional response and associations. Sure, you might know that this kind of work can greatly reduce or eliminate your pain, but without practice, your emotions may be caught behind. A lot of negative emotional baggage comes with chronic pain, and it will take dedicated practice to untangle it. Practice it until it becomes automatic. It's like how a pilot clocks up hours upon hours in a controlled simulator environment; when disaster strikes, their response is automatic and unconscious. The same goes for this work. Practice it in a controlled environment so that when something bad happens, all the practice kicks into gear without a second thought. Building this habit short circuits willpower and self-control.

Starting unfamiliar, emotionally difficult tasks—like somatic tracking—invites **procrastination**. Procrastination looks like wanting to read more material, post in a support group, or watch a pain-related video without actually putting it to use. It feels like you are doing pain management "work," but you are just consuming information without necessarily spending time out of your day to practice it. Time spent here is not time spent healing. The research-based method of overcoming procrastination is to resolve the underlying feeling of fear or sadness. Ask yourself: What specifically is making me fearful?

Another method to help overcome procrastination is to start tiny—say with 30 seconds of practice. Set yourself a goal and commitment to not read another book or article until you have spent several weeks implementing the last one. Reward yourself with some social media only after your 10-minute timer has gone off. Instead of taking time to read more material, take time to complete some somatic tracking or journaling.

When my recovery "wasn't working" or I felt like "nothing was happening," I would get **frustrated by the theory**. This gives rise to an important question: What happens when you have a deep intellectual insight and head knowledge that does not produce change? This seems somewhat counterintuitive because if neuroplastic pain is a tricky creation of the mind, surely better knowledge in our mind will help displace it. If we squeeze another book's worth of material in, our "bad" concept of pain will be squeezed out, right? One in, one out. Good for bad.

But pain is an experience. So is somatic tracking. By now, you have picked up that **experiencing** is necessary for the therapeutic effect. Experiencing an event is different from knowing a bit of information. Experiencing and knowing are not synonymous. Experience conjures words of "involvement," "sensing," and "participation," whereas knowing brings up the idea of "intelligence" or "insight." Somatic tracking is experiencing. You cannot intellectualize an experience. You can't research your way out of experiencing. It has to be felt in the body. This means jumping in and doing it. This is why consistent routine and practice are essential, rewarding, and ultimately satisfying. We treat pain with an experience.

Feeling like you're **not making progress** in managing chronic pain is common. Remember, chronic pain management is a habit, and habits take weeks and months to properly set in place. Forcing a timeframe on you can also be counterintuitive. From the outset, it is not possible to put a calendar date on when you will feel better, so why burden yourself with a deadline that is only artificial and will likely cause more grief than anything else? I am not saying that you shouldn't check in and reassess your progress every now and then. The ultimate aim should be the practice of these proven techniques rather than instantaneous healing. Just like sustainable dieting shouldn't have a goal of hitting a target weight quickly (which tempts you with crash diets and unhealthy eating, which may cause rebound), but rather consistent, measured, healthy eating and exercise day in, day out. Weight loss is just a side effect.

For those who are still stuck, maybe you are **not doing the task** to help reduce pain. It's easy to overlook things or not be 100% clear on how to start the task. Revisiting the relevant sections of this book is the first step. If you are not doing your practice, the next step is to reduce the time commitment—like changing a 10-minute writing session into just "getting out your pen and paper" or finding a single trigger. Make it as small as humanly possible, so you maximize your ability to stick with it.

Finally, if you are still feeling stuck, you can send me an email (sam@pastpainbook.com) and I will do my best to clarify things. This book was designed to get you *unstuck*, and if you are still feeling unsure about what to do next, I would love to help you out.

Your takeaways from Chapter 7

Somatic tracking is the best-proven method for reducing neuroplastic pain. It's a psychological intervention that decouples physical pain sensations from our emotions. This changes how our brain responds when faced with pain.

The crux of pain management is being able to default to somatic tracking when you notice a pain trigger or flare-up. Increase your skills by:

- Improving your vocabulary around pain. Better descriptor words assist in tracking.
- Practice by noticing your breath or scanning your body. Don't try to change anything; just notice what happens.
- Undertake advanced somatic tracking by locating where the pain occurs and observing and describing how it changes in location or quality.
- Reappraise the "terrible pain" into "just one of many different bodily sensations."

Afterword

The scariest thing that happened to me

Chronic pain was the worst thing that happened in my life. The pain in my wrists and arms was excruciating. It was paralyzing during a flare-up. During a lull period, I used to fear it all the time. Eventually, I used to fear the thought of fearing it. It had spiraled out of control.

This is all to say that I wasn't very good at managing my pain.

But then something happened that scared me more. My pain started getting just a tiny bit... better. My gut reaction was to assume that my mind was playing tricks on me. It was such a minute difference that I was afraid to admit it to myself in case I jinxed it or stopped it in its tracks. I (stupidly) hid it from my doctors in case I was wrong about the turning of the tide after all.

It's OK to celebrate these momentary periods of relief, even if they are small and fleeting.

Practicing the steps in this book helped me to the point of recovery. And what got me to this point is letting go of the idea of a finish line or calendar date. The goal here is to build a system that inevitably erodes your pain.

Together, we've seen that effective pain management doesn't have to be serendipitous. We can design it in a way that is simple to implement, effective at reducing pain severity (from seven out of ten to three out of ten), and durable, so you won't be left shipwrecked if a setback occurs.

Remember that neuroplastic pain is primarily psychological, and pain's sneakiest trick is stealing your focus away from your mind and back on your physical body.

You've learned three (potentially unconventional) ideas about building a pain management system:

1. Releasing emotions and stressors through **writing**. This lets you step back and look at things objectively, as if reading a case study on somebody else.
2. Instead of ruminating and festering on past flare-ups, use them as an opportunity to note things that **trigger** pain. Plans can be made to eliminate or reduce these triggers to keep one step ahead of the pain cycle.

3. If you feel stuck, or unsure of what to do next, it's probably a sign to do 10 minutes of **somatic tracking**. Amplify your curiosity and self-compassion of your body's signals and try playing with some new descriptor words for pain, like "tingling," "discomfort," "itching," or "sensation."

Everything in this book has been designed for, and tested with, neuroplastic pain sufferers. It might seem like an information overload, but these small steps are totally achievable. The action for you to take now is to carve out that precious 10 minutes of your day and just start, even if it's not perfect. With repetition, this management system will become automatic.

What recovery looks like

Treating neuroplastic pain is a journey, and there are plenty of guideposts to indicate you are heading in the right direction, even if it doesn't feel that way at the time. Things to celebrate include:

- setting a goal to reduce pain to a three out of ten
- finishing your first writing session
- forming a hypothesis about what a trigger might be
- the lightbulb moment of identifying a trigger you hadn't noticed before

- completing your first attempt at somatic tracking
- sitting with a difficult sensation and describing it with different adjectives
- putting 10 minutes of effort in, even on a day that you don't feel like "showing up"
- finding counter-evidence of times you are not in pain
- recovering from a derailment or big life interruption
- performing a physical movement that previously would have caused pain without being in pain.

Finally, what does recovery look like? That's a question best answered by the many early readers of this book who've shared their perspectives. I hope you find these as encouraging as I did:

- "Feeling like I am in control, not the pain. A change of tide. Empowerment."
- "Self-identifying as 'functionally recovered.'"
- "Not being bothered by pain anymore because I know how to deal with it if it flares up."
- "Surprising my physician at a recent visit."
- "Recommencing hobbies I had to give up."
- "Learning to say 'no' to people."
- "Having a deeper sense of calm and self-compassion."

- "Friends and family commenting that I 'seem happier' or 'look different.'"
- "Being excited, not fearful, about the future."

Acknowledgments

Thank you to the almost 100 early readers and supporters who were incredibly generous with their time, insights, beta reading, and feedback. This alone improved this book out of sight and helped me on my mission to make pain management a little bit better. Given the nature of neuroplastic pain, few elected to publish their names. I thank Carrie Martin, Capi, Kalli O'Connor, Nathanael Horton, and Scott McEwan. The rest of you know who you are—so thanks.

A big shout out to my writing buddies over at the Useful Author's community: Clare Treson, Leanne Hughes, KimSia Sim, and Brian McCann. Thanks for helping me keep up the writing momentum.

Thank you to my parents, Graeme and Jane, whose unconditional support built the foundation for this successful yet meandering recovery journey.

And, finally, to Ali whose support and encouragement enabled me to complete this book.

Thanks and next steps

I really appreciate you taking the leap of faith and spending a few hours of your precious time reading this guide.

Please shoot me an email (sam@pastpainbook.com) to let me know how you're getting on with your pain management. I'd love to hear about it.

One final request from me. Could you take two minutes right now to leave a review at the place you purchased this from? It doesn't have to be super-polished—a few words are totally fine (the fastest way to an independent author's heart is through a review). You can think of this as a gift to future readers.

Wishing you all the very best,
Sam Evans

Bibliography

Apkarian, A. V., Hashmi, J. A., & Baliki, M. N. (2011). Pain and the brain: specificity and plasticity of the brain in clinical chronic pain. *Pain, 152*(3), S49-S64.

Ashar, Y. K., Chang, L. J., & Wager, T. D. (2017). Brain mechanisms of the placebo effect: an affective appraisal account. *Annual review of clinical psychology, 13*, 73-98.

Ashar, Y. K., Gordon, A., Schubiner, H., Uipi, C., Knight, K., Anderson, Z., Carlisle, J., Polisky, L., Geuter, S., Flood, T. F. & Kragel, P. A. (2022). Effect of pain reprocessing therapy vs placebo and usual care for patients with chronic back pain: a randomized clinical trial. *JAMA psychiatry 79*.1 (2022): 13-23.

Asmundson, G. J., & Katz, J. (2009). Understanding the co-occurrence of anxiety disorders and chronic pain: state-of-the-art. *Depression and anxiety, 26*(10), 888-901.

Bayer, T. L., Baer, P. E., & Early, C. (1991). Situational and psychophysiological factors in psychologically induced pain. *Pain, 44*(1), 45-50.

Begley, S. (2007). *Train your mind, change your brain: How a new science reveals our extraordinary potential to transform ourselves* (Vol. 214). Ballantine Books.

Bernhard, T. (2018). *How to be sick: A Buddhist-inspired guide for the chronically ill and their caregivers.* Simon and Schuster.

Boersma, K., & Linton, S. J. (2006). Expectancy, fear and pain in the prediction of chronic pain and disability: a prospective analysis. *European Journal of Pain, 10*(6), 551-557.

Broom, B. (1997). *Somatic illness and the patient's other story: a practical integrative mind/body approach to disease for doctors and psychotherapists.* London: Free Association Books.

Broom, B. (2018). *Meaning-full disease: How personal experience and meanings cause and maintain physical illness.* Routledge.

Carty, J. N., Ziadni, M. S., Holmes, H. J., Tomakowsky, J., Peters, K., Schubiner, H., & Lumley, M. A. (2019). The effects of a life stress emotional awareness and expression interview for women with chronic urogenital pain: a randomized controlled trial. *Pain medicine, 20*(7), 1321-1329.

Castro, W. H. M., Meyer, S. J., Becke, M. E. R., Nentwig, C. G., Hein, M. F., Ercan, B. I., Thomann, S., Wessels, U., & Du Chesne, A. E. (2001). No stress—no whiplash? Prevalence of "whiplash" symptoms following exposure to a placebo rear-end collision. *International journal of legal medicine, 114*, 316-322.

Clarke, D. D. (2007). *They can't find anything wrong!: 7 keys to understanding, treating, and healing stress illness.* Sentient Publications.

Clarke, D. D., Schubiner, H., Clark-Smith, M., & Abbass, A. (Eds.). (2019). *Psychophysiologic disorders: Trauma informed, interprofessional diagnosis and treatment.* Psychophysiologic Disorders Association.

Craig, A. D. (2003). Interoception: the sense of the physiological condition of the body. *Current opinion in neurobiology, 13*(4), 500-505.

Critchley, H. D., Wiens, S., Rotshtein, P., Öhman, A., & Dolan, R. J. (2004). Neural systems supporting interoceptive awareness. *Nature neuroscience, 7*(2), 189-195.

Doidge, N. (2007). *The brain that changes itself: Stories of personal triumph from the frontiers of brain science.* Penguin.

Doll, A., Hölzel, B. K., Bratec, S. M., Boucard, C. C., Xie, X., Wohlschläger, A. M., & Sorg, C. (2016). Mindful attention to breath regulates emotions via increased amygdala–prefrontal cortex connectivity. *Neuroimage, 134*, 305-313.

Donnino, M. W., Thompson, G. S., Mehta, S., Paschali, M., Howard, P., Antonsen, S. B., Balaji, L., Bertisch, S. M., Edwards, R., Ngo, L. H., & Grossestreuer, A. V. (2021). Psychophysiologic symptom relief therapy for chronic back pain: a pilot randomized controlled trial. *Pain Reports, 6*(3).

Engel, G. L. (1977). The need for a new medical model: a challenge for biomedicine. *Science, 196*(4286), 129-136.

Engert, V., Smallwood, J., & Singer, T. (2014). Mind your thoughts: Associations between self-generated thoughts and stress-induced and baseline levels of cortisol and alpha-amylase. *Biological psychology, 103*, 283-291.

Fogg, B. J. (2009). A behavior model for persuasive design. In *Proceedings of the 4th International Conference on Persuasive Technology* (pp. 1-7).

Bibliography

Gordon, A., & Ziv, A. (2021). *The way out: A revolutionary, scientifically proven approach to healing chronic pain.* Penguin.

Gracely, R. H., Geisser, M. E., Giesecke, T., Grant, M. A. B., Petzke, F., Williams, D. A., & Clauw, D. J. (2004). Pain catastrophizing and neural responses to pain among persons with fibromyalgia. *Brain, 127*(4), 835-843.

Graham, J. E., Lobel, M., Glass, P., & Lokshina, I. (2008). Effects of written anger expression in chronic pain patients: making meaning from pain. *Journal of behavioral medicine, 31,* 201-212.

Gupta, A., Silman, A. J., Ray, D., Morriss, R., Dickens, C., MacFarlane, G. J., Chiu, Y. H., Nicholl, B., & McBeth, J. (2007). The role of psychosocial factors in predicting the onset of chronic widespread pain: results from a prospective population-based study. *Rheumatology, 46*(4), 666-671.

Harvie, D. S., Moseley, G. L., Hillier, S. L., & Meulders, A. (2017). Classical conditioning differences associated with chronic pain: a systematic review. *The Journal of Pain, 18*(8), 889-898.

Hsu, M. C., Schubiner, H., Lumley, M. A., Stracks, J. S., Clauw, D. J., & Williams, D. A. (2010). Sustained pain reduction through affective self-awareness in fibromyalgia: a randomized controlled trial. *Journal of General Internal Medicine, 25,* 1064-1070.

Jensen, M. C., Brant-Zawadzki, M. N., Obuchowski, N., Modic, M. T., Malkasian, D., & Ross, J. S. (1994). Magnetic resonance imaging of the lumbar spine in people without back pain. *New England Journal of Medicine, 331*(2), 69-73.

Khoo, E. L., Small, R., Cheng, W., Hatchard, T., Glynn, B., Rice, D. B., Skidmore, B., Kenny, S., Hutton, B., & Poulin, P. A. (2019). Comparative evaluation of group-based mindfulness-based stress reduction and cognitive behavioural therapy for the treatment and management of chronic pain: A systematic review and network meta-analysis. *BMJ Ment Health, 22*(1), 26-35.

Kuner, R., & Flor, H. (2017). Structural plasticity and reorganisation in chronic pain. *Nature Reviews Neuroscience, 18*(1), 20-30.

Lumley, M. A., Cohen, J. L., Borszcz, G. S., Cano, A., Radcliffe, A. M., Porter, L. S., Schubiner, H., & Keefe, F. J. (2011). Pain and emotion: a biopsychosocial review of recent research. *Journal of clinical psychology, 67*(9), 942-968.

Lumley, M. A., & Schubiner, H. (2019). Emotional awareness and expression therapy for chronic pain: Rationale, principles and techniques, evidence, and critical review. *Current rheumatology reports, 21*, 1-8.

Maté, G. (2011). *When the body says no: The cost of hidden stress.* Vintage Canada.

McCroskey, J. C., Daly, J. A., & Sorensen, G. (1976). Personality correlates of communication apprehension: A research note. *Human Communication Research, 2*(4), 376-380.

Melzack, R., Coderre, T. J., Katz, J., & Vaccarino, A. L. (2001). Central neuroplasticity and pathological pain. *Annals of the New York Academy of Sciences, 933*(1), 157-174.

Minton, K., Ogden, P., & Pain, C. (2006). *Trauma and the body: A sensorimotor approach to psychotherapy (Norton series on interpersonal neurobiology).* WW Norton & Company.

Moseley, G. L. (2007). Reconceptualising pain according to modern pain science. *Physical therapy reviews, 12*(3), 169-178.

Payne, H., & Brooks, S. D. (2017). Moving on: the BodyMind approach for medically unexplained symptoms. *Journal of public mental health, 16*(2), 63-71.

Picavet, H. S. J., Vlaeyen, J. W., & Schouten, J. S. (2002). Pain catastrophizing and kinesiophobia: predictors of chronic low back pain. *American journal of epidemiology, 156*(11), 1028-1034.

Raja, S. N., Carr, D. B., Cohen, M., Finnerup, N. B., Flor, H., Gibson, S., Keefe, F. J., Mogil, J. S., Ringkamp, M., Sluka, K. A., & Song, X. J. (2020). The revised International Association for the Study of Pain definition of pain: concepts, challenges, and compromises. *Pain, 161*(9), 1976-1982.

Samwel, H. J., Kraaimaat, F. W., Evers, A. W., & Crul, B. J. (2007). The role of fear-avoidance and helplessness in explaining functional disability in chronic pain: a prospective study. *International Journal of Behavioral Medicine, 14*, 237-241.

Sarno, J. E. (2011). *The divided mind: The epidemic of mindbody disorders.* Prelude Books.

Schubiner, H., & Betzold, M. (2010). Unlearn your pain. *Pleasant Ridge, MI: Mind Body Publishing.*

Siegel, D. J. (2009). Mindful awareness, mindsight, and neural integration. *The Humanistic Psychologist, 37*(2), 137-158.

Siegel, D. J. (2012). *Mindsight: Change your brain and your life.* Scribe Publications.

Sirois, F. M. (2022). *Procrastination: What it is, why it's a problem, and what you can do about it.* American Psychological Association.

Smart, K. M. (2023). The biopsychosocial model of pain in physiotherapy: past, present and future. *Physical Therapy Reviews,* 1-10.

Tankha, H., Lumley, M. A., Gordon, A., Schubiner, H., Uipi, C., Harris, J., Wager, T. D., & Ashar, Y. K. (2023). "I don't have chronic back pain anymore": Patient Experiences in Pain Reprocessing Therapy for Chronic Back Pain. *The Journal of Pain.*

Tracey, I. (2010). Getting the pain you expect: mechanisms of placebo, nocebo and reappraisal effects in humans. *Nature medicine, 16*(11), 1277-1283.

Van der Kolk, B. (2014). The body keeps the score: Brain, mind, and body in the healing of trauma.

Woo, C. W., Schmidt, L., Krishnan, A., Jepma, M., Roy, M., Lindquist, M. A., Atlas, L. Y., & Wager, T. D. (2017). Quantifying cerebral contributions to pain beyond nociception. *Nature communications, 8*(1), 14211.

Woolf, C. J. (2011). Central sensitization: implications for the diagnosis and treatment of pain. *Pain, 152*(3), S2-S15.

Yarns, B. C., Lumley, M. A., Cassidy, J. T., Steers, W. N., Osato, S., Schubiner, H., & Sultzer, D. L. (2020). Emotional awareness and expression therapy achieves greater pain reduction than cognitive behavioral therapy in older adults with chronic musculoskeletal pain: a preliminary randomized comparison trial. *Pain Medicine, 21*(11), 2811-2822.

Printed in Dunstable, United Kingdom